For the Record:

My Life as a Heart and

Chest Surgeon

By George C. Heitzman, MD

1/30/2010
Dear Tom
Thank you so much
for attending this seminar
wish the best-
George

First Paperback printing, December 2010
Printed in the United States of America

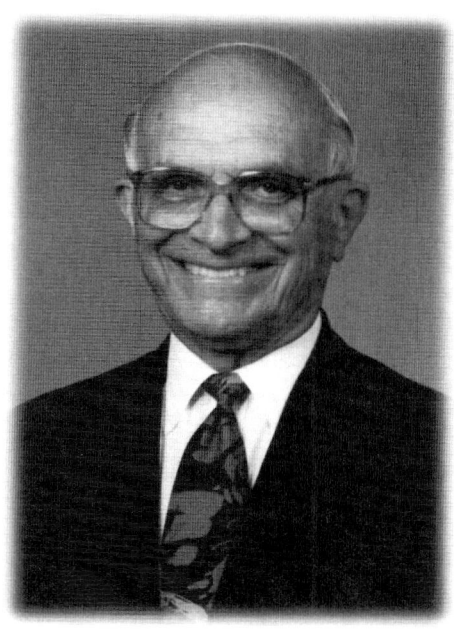

This book is dedicated to my one and only brother,
the late Dr. Edward James Heitzman,
alias Jim or E.J.
He was my hero.
His untimely death on November 11, 1996,
was a huge loss to me.

It is also my intent to remember my many patients,
whom I have loved,
and who have been such a joy over the years.

Chapter One

FOR THE RECORD

After retiring from private practice in chest surgery in 1988, I began reflecting on many incidents in my career and considered writing a book about them. I kept putting it off until 2008, when a pleasant surprise occurred.

Out of nowhere, my brother's daughter, Dr. Karen Heitzman, an outstanding internist practicing in Syracuse, relayed a fax received from Joe Palmieri. He was a former patient of mine who wanted to talk with me and obtain his medical records from 39 years ago. It seems that at age 80, most of his friends were no longer alive and yet he was going strong, despite a big open heart operation in 1969. The hospital involved, St. Joseph's, no longer had his records, but I have kept all of my heart surgery cases since performing the first open heart operation in Syracuse in November, 1958. Having retired 20 years ago, I had shredded most of my patient's charts earlier in the year, except for the heart surgery cases. These were the earliest open heart operations performed in Syracuse and represented medical history. Fortunately, Joe's chart was retrieved without difficulty and I faxed him copies of the operative report and heart catheterization.

I reviewed the details in his record and they were amazing.

Palmieri's father died of heart disease in his 50s. Joe had his first and subsequent "coronaries" during his 30s. He was treated at the local VA hospital as an in-patient for several months. Prior to discharge, he was told he had a "bubble" on his heart but no specific treatment was recommended. He continued to work and at age 42, consulted his cousin and family physician, Dr. Paul Maglione, of North Syracuse. After examining him, Paul immediately referred him to the Msgr. Toomey Cardiopulmonary and Research Laboratory at St. Joseph's Hospital and its director, Dr. Goffredo Gensini. Joe underwent a heart catheterization the next day and a large aneurysm of the left ventricle was found containing the usual thrombus (clot). Joe was referred to my brother, internist-cardiologist, Dr. Edward J. Heitzman and then to me, for surgery. His wife was pregnant and we postponed surgery for a month until she delivered.

On June 4, 1969, open heart surgery employing the Mayo-Gibbons heart-lung was carried out and the aneurysm removed. His coronary arteries surprisingly showed no significant obstructive disease. Therefore, no other procedure was required. Joe's post-operative course was uneventful and the last office visit 11 months later was very satisfactory. He moved out of Syracuse two years after surgery and continued to do very well and remain active, except for recently requiring a cardiac pacemaker.

Sensing he might be an unusual statistic, Joe contacted me to try to research this further.

The case was most unusual to have suffered such a big "blow-out" of the left ventricle and survive without its bursting, not to mention living into his 80s without requiring subsequent surgery.

He contacted the American Heart Association about his medical history and more specific data was requested. Even his own physician questioned his story of an aneurysm removed so many years before and his still living at age 80. As he coyly responded, "I know I had the surgery because I have the scar to prove it."

Since our first telephone conversation, Joe and I never stopped communicating. His class reunion at Ithaca College, Ithaca, New York, was held in June 2008 and he asked if I would meet him there, 60 miles from Syracuse. My wife, Gina, and I decided late Friday evening that we would drive to Ithaca College the following day to meet him.

Joe had been editor of the college newspaper and knows his way around. Two reporters and a photographer were waiting for this meeting. It was truly a heartfelt reunion. A lovely photo and article made the front page of the local

Ithaca newspaper. It was evident there was a special chemistry between us.

This reached the Syracuse newspaper, and another front page story—"To Touch Hearts"--appeared. Since then, the phone calls and emails have been constant.

It would be safe to say things have not been the same since hearing from Joey last March. The idea of writing about my experiences has become a priority. The need for this book is not for personal "accolades." I received that fulfillment through the years from my work.

I do feel it is extremely important to document history and give credit to where it is due.

My patients are my validation.

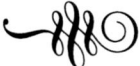

To protect their privacy, all patients are referred to by initials only. I have used actual names in cases that were reported on by the media, and thus are already part of the public record.

Chapter Two

THE EARLY YEARS

My brother Jim and I had a wonderful childhood and life-long relationship. He was one year younger and we shared the same bedroom with twin beds for 24 years before leaving for internship together for two more years. Along with our parents, Katharine Cook Heitzman and George James Andrew Heitzman, we lived in a two-family house with mom's parents, Mamie and Jake. Our son Jake was named in his honor. (We never called them anything else.) Being the only children in the family, Jim and I received much attention from Jake's three sisters, Aunts Frankie, Kate, and Clara, along with her husband Frank Snyder, a retired pharmacist who lived across the street. As youngsters we were constantly with them. Aunt Frankie owned a cottage on Oneida Lake. She and Kate spent summers there and Jim and I stayed with them. It was truly paradise, with the best food, swimming, fishing and boating available. Jake would come down during the week and our parents on the weekends.

In school, we were good students and played sports at East Syracuse High School. Jim was by far the better athlete. He was an all-county quarterback and linebacker in football and once played a game with his arm strapped to his side. He was one tough guy!

Our mother had a profound influence on us in subtle ways. As a registered nurse, she had a medical orientation. We were raised from an early age wanting to be doctors and had a special relationship with our own family doctor, Ray Seagfried; Jim and I even received Christmas presents from him.

We saw Dad's only brother and his family only on occasion as they were not in close proximity. His son, Dr. Robert Heitzman, became professor and head of the department of radiology at Upstate Medical Center. He is internationally known and author of a text on tomography of the chest, which I have been miscredited for on occasion!

Dad's three sisters lived together in Syracuse. One was married to an inventor, Joe Sheboe, and the other two lived with them. Joe also had a radio store but, for some reason, my parents never did business with him. Once or twice a year, the four of them would visit us unannounced. When we spotted them through the front window we would rush and move the huge radio console in the living room into the back so they wouldn't see it. It was rather humorous afterwards, but, certainly not at the time.

Uncle Joe was also quite a fisherman and story teller. He would describe fishing on the St. Lawrence to us and this seemed quite sophisticated compared to our Oneida Lake experiences. Once when Jim and I were in our early teens, Uncle Joe came down to Oneida Lake to fish. We were very excited. He arrived in the early morning and had all sorts of equipment. We did supply the crabs he wanted and the three of us set out in our small aluminum boat with a five-horsepower Neptune engine. Jim and I planned to take him to our favorite bar in the middle of the lake, three miles away. He had other plans and wanted to fish off-shore, just around nearby Shackleton's Point (now a research area for Cornell University). We had passed the area hundreds of times but never fished there, thinking it was not worthwhile.

Jim and I looked at each other, visualizing a lousy day of fishing. Uncle Joe picked the spot to fish, an area 20 feet offshore, in three feet of water. We cringed, but obliged. Within an hour we had caught the limit of good-size small-mouth bass. Uncle Joe said nothing, as he had expected these super results but Jim and I were in shock.

Before he left, Uncle Joe gave us the beautiful live fish net that was used that amazing morning. It was the greatest fishing I ever experienced but, may not have been for my brother who went on to become a great fisherman who caught literally thousands. (He always threw them back, unless we were fishing together and if I wanted to keep them, he would oblige.)

Uncle Joe never called to return and fish again. He was a very wise man and knew when he was ahead.

In later years, near the end of our medical careers, Jim and I fished together off Captiva Island, Florida, where he had a time-share condo. Our guide, Captain Fisher, was aptly named and extremely accommodating. The gulf scene was breathtaking and included schools of dolphins and manatees.

Captain Fisher's 30-foot-boat on the Gulf of Mexico was a far cry from our early days in our infamous aluminum boat on Oneida Lake. We were always successful catching grouper and this became my favorite entree choice. On one trip, our great friend and former classmate, the late Dr. Jerry Segal (a radiologist originally from Utica, then living in Naples, Florida) was aboard. He and I sat in front with E.J. and Jake in the stern. The captain cautioned us to always hold our fishing poles and never set them down. After some quiet minutes, Jerry placed his pole nearby and we lost track of it. Suddenly, we watched the pole slip out of the boat into the gulf. We were all stunned but the good-natured Captain Fisher was furious. We were fishing in approximately 30 feet of choppy water and the anchored boat was swinging back and forth over a width of approximately 50 feet. We all knew there was no chance of retrieving the expensive pole and were saddened to say the least. After about 15 minutes I felt my line tug and asked the captain to help reel in my catch. He obliged and suddenly his disgusted expression changed into one of total pleasure as he yelled, "You caught my pole!" and reeled in Jerry's pole.

Thereafter, all was well and a great fishing day ended with a lovely catered dinner by South Seas Plantation, including linens and silver courtesy of Jim and B.C. Heitzman.

Even into his sixties, Jim was a fine, physical specimen who lifted weights daily and was known to go para-sailing on Captiva.

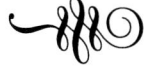

Chapter Three

THE CAREFREE YEARS

Having graduated from East Syracuse High School in 1941, I attended Syracuse University in the pre-med program. My brother did the same, starting one year later. We both received early acceptance to Syracuse medical school, then owned by Syracuse University. Jim had two years of pre-med and me three when we started. We were probably the only two brothers in the same class in the school's history. I made Phi Beta Kappa and Jim likely would have if he had more pre-med preparation.

After admittance we were taken into the military service, Jim in the Army, and me in the Navy. During my physical exam, the medical officer (actually a dentist) found my blood pressure too high on two occasions. Before the third and final exam, the corpsman told me to take deep breaths just beforehand. (Hyperventilation results in eliminating carbon dioxide with a resultant drop in blood pressure. I found this out later in school.) It worked and I passed.

In medical school, we studied and worked very hard as the program was accelerated into three years instead of four. Our class was heterogeneous indeed. Ages varied from 21 to over 50 on admission. One student I knew from pre-med at Syracuse was a "classical playboy" with connections. Another was in his 50s and my pre-med advisor at Syracuse University. Admittedly these were huge surprises on opening day.

The students were in part selected by the military services and came from throughout the United States and Puerto Rico. A class of 58 started, including three female students--a marked contrast to today's medical school classes of 150, half of whom are women.

The atmosphere was far from congenial with our faculty with few exceptions. Although we were not on active duty, we were being prepared as military physicians and received military pay. There was probably resentment because our income was as great as some of theirs.

The mortality at the end of two years was 33 percent. These cuts were made without warning. As class president, I went to the dean, a nationally known figure in academic medical circles, but never received a satisfactory explanation. A number of physician's sons failed out, and as it turned out, the dean's own son failed and then became a New York forest ranger.

Some felt there was also inequity in the selection process for honors students to be admitted to the Alpha Omega Alpha honors fraternity. Most were solid choices by far. However, the pre-med playboy with connections was selected, as was my pre-med advisor at Syracuse University. The latter was a charmer and had one female professor so influenced that when her examination asked for specific drug dosages he put down 1 tablet, 2 tablets, etc. without using grams or other specific values and was given an A.

Despite the politics and tremendous workload, these were the most carefree days of my life. There was much camaraderie. We had our weekend beer parties at one of the two fraternity houses, Nu Sigma Nu and Alpha Kappa Kappa and this was our stress relief.

We also played sports. My hero came through when we were playing an undergraduate fraternity for the intramural championship in basketball at Syracuse University. It was a spirited game and an opponent and I were about to come to blows when, out of nowhere, someone grabbed this big fellow from behind and promptly deposited him firmly but, gently on the floor, rendering him totally helpless and ending the altercation. It was my brother, Jim! We won that game and had some outstanding athletes on the team.

One of my buddies was classmate Mario Prioletti. In pre-med, he had taken many psychology courses, including hypnosis. We all thought he would become a psychiatrist. In the anatomy lab, the large room was filled with cadavers each on a table with walking spaces between them. On occasion

"Prio" would hypnotize the smartest student in the class, Henry Ludeman, and we would parade him past the cadavers. His body was rigid and he would be carried by his head and heels. Fortunately, Dr. Armstrong, professor of anatomy, either never saw this or was roaring in his office.

In our second year, four of us went to the hospital to watch an operation for the first time. Up until then, all of our medical education was didactic and we had absolutely no hospital exposure. The observatory was glassed in and we therefore were partitioned from the operating room itself. The procedure we observed was a hernia repair. It was so quiet you could hear a pin drop. Once the incision was made through the skin and blood appeared, three of us heard a loud thud. The fourth observer had fainted! He ultimately became one of the busiest surgeons in Syracuse and we used to razz him often about that day.

At commencement, Jim and I had the honor of leading the entire Syracuse University graduating class into the old Archbold Stadium. Our parents were thrilled. Subsequently, this structure was torn down and replaced with the now famous Carrier Dome

A large number of our graduating classmates never once returned for a class reunion. Nevertheless it is my strong conviction that I received a fine medical school education and that both Jim and I were very well prepared for future hospital training. Never once did we feel inferior to our fellow interns from Harvard, Yale, Cornell, Columbia, or University of Pennsylvania, etc.

Chapter Four

IN TRAINING

In the continuing spirit of togetherness, Jim and I went on and interned for two years at the Rhode Island Hospital in Providence, R.I. It was excellent training and we each discovered our areas of specialty--Jim in medicine and I in surgery.

Jim became famous for his ambulance rides to ships in the nearby Narragansett Harbor to retrieve injured personnel. A movie was made of this and shown in a local theatre. The main actor was "the intern with the horned-rim glasses," my brother. It was a hit.

I decided to become a surgeon largely because of the wonderful way I was treated, especially by a senior staff surgeon, Dr. Robert Baldridge. He was a fine surgeon, Harvard and Boston trained, and quite demanding. He took a liking to me and would say to the surgical resident, "Why don't you let George do that hernia?" It was quite embarrassing, but I got to do a lot.

I still remember caring for A. Q., a young man about my age, with severe second- and third-degree burns over much of his body. This was before the use of potassium was known and the mortality of such an injury was very high. I spent many hours caring for A., changing his dressings, etc. We also used infant's foreskins from nearby Lying-In Obstetrical Hospital to temporarily cover the burn sites until his own skin grafts took over.

The fellow interns were great guys and I cannot recall a "bad apple." Dick Hornberger was from Maine and a Cornell graduate. He was very quiet and difficult to get to know. Dick was also in the straight surgical internship the second year and I never knew where he went after. Years later, the television hit *Mash* became everyone's favorite and I learned that Hornberger wrote the story while stationed in Korea. He actually was "Hawkeye." I did see him once at a chest meeting in Toronto and we talked briefly. He is undoubtedly one of the wealthiest doctors I have ever met or at least one of the most famous interns I have worked with.

In this era, good internships paid no salaries and this was so at Rhode Island. We were given our uniforms, meals, and a daily beverage, including beer. We were all hurting for money and our parents were generous. Some of the guys would hoard the beer for a few weeks and then "party!"

During my internship on the urology service, I had some unusual cases. One in particular was a male in his 20s who presented in the emergency room with a glass swizzle rod broken off in his penis. In a serious manner, he explained that he and his girlfriend were having drinks and by chance this had slipped out of his hand and dropped into his penis! That was our entertainment for the evening.

During the second year of my internship I had my first paper published in *the Rhode Island Medical Journal,* "A Review of the Treatment of Peripheral Arteriosclerotic Disease."

In retrospect, the field of vascular disease had always interested me. I also was fascinated by the work of Drs. Shute from Canada and their studies connecting vitamin E (tocopherols) as essential ingredients of our vascular system. All of my life I have been a strong advocate of nutrition and many of these are now known as anti-oxidants.

In 1949, brother Jim and I split to follow our chosen fields. He had very fine training in Boston at the Boston City Hospital and Pratt Diagnostic. I went to New York City for one year in pathology at St. Luke's Hospital, affiliated with Columbia Medical Center.

In 1950, Jim was taken into the military. He joined the Airborne, which is one tough assignment. He trained at its center at Fort Campbell, Kentucky, and was then shipped to California. There his sweetheart nurse from the Rhode Island Hospital, B.C. Larson, and he were married and thereafter spent over four decades of a wonderful life together.

Fortunately, he never left for Korea. After two years in

the service, he returned to Boston to complete his training in internal medicine. Although promised a residency in cardiology at the Rhode Island Hospital, it never materialized. He said nothing, but I knew it was extremely disappointing. He was a very strong man in every sense.

Jim returned to Syracuse to private practice in internal medicine. For a period he was Medical Director at St. Joseph's Hospital.

My year in pathology at St. Luke's was great, but I realized that this was not the field for me. Residencies in surgery were in great demand and returning doctors from active military service were given first choice. I applied to the Syracuse Medical Center, now owned by New York State. At the interview, the chief of surgery, Dr. Arthur Raffl, told me he would give me his decision in a few days. That very day, Dr. Joe Delmonico, an excellent attending anesthesiologist, overheard Dr. Raffl say that I was accepted and immediately called to give me the good news. I shall never forget his kindness. Joe was the brother of surgeon Ernie Delmonico, Sr., who would play a major role in my story in later years.

While a surgical resident at Upstate Medical Center 1950-1953, I experienced an event not fully appreciated until years later. For some reason I was appointed to give a tour to a prospective first-ever full time Director of Surgery at Upstate, Dr. Norman Shumway. He was my age and very pleasant in all respects. I was given very little information about him, but looking over the surgical physical layout he said something I shall never forget: "I would have no room for my monkey colony"!

It was another way of saying "Syracuse does not have what I need."

Shumway went on to continue with his surgical training at the National Institute of Health and the University of Minnesota under the legendary Dr. Owen Wangensteen who was well known to train outstanding academic surgeons. Shumway is correctly credited for the pioneering and development of cardiac transplantation there and at Standord Medical Center, Palo Alto, California and is considered the father of cardiac transplantation.

I shall never forget this meeting with one of the greats in cardiac surgery and research.

I preferred and was allowed to spend most of my time at St. Joseph's Hospital, as it was part of the medical center rotation. I enjoyed the attendings there, especially Dr. Charles Demong. Chuck was about 10 years my senior. He was a Syracuse native, having graduated from Syracuse University and medical school. He trained surgically at the Mayo Clinic as a fellow and was then taken into the military and assigned to Fitzsimmons Army Hospital, in Denver. This was the center for all major military thoracic injuries and the chief of surgery was regular Army Colonel John Grow, MD. The experience there was phenomenal. After discharge from the Army, Chuck returned to Syracuse to practice general and thoracic surgery, and was board certified in both.

He was particularly good to me and provided much surgical experience. In addition to the surgeries, I was allowed to care for his office practice if he was away for a day, a trust and responsibility I have never heard of before or since. He was an excellent surgeon and a great physical specimen who used to walk around the operating room on his hands. Say no more!

In 1952, there was a surgical meeting in New York City where Dr. Demong met his old chief, Dr. John Groon, who offered him partnership in his private surgery practice in Denver. Grow had left the military and was an immediate success in the Mile High City. Chuck's wife did not care for Syracuse and this may have been a big factor in his leaving.

At the same time, I was due to enter the military. I was very interested in chest surgery and Dr. Demong told me there was a thoracic surgical residency program at the National Jewish Hospital in Denver, under the direction of Grow. He would arrange for me to be selected resident there on finishing military service in 1955.

While he moved back to Denver, I spent two years in the Army at La Rochelle, France, located between Paris and

Bourdeaux, performing substantial surgeries. This was an excellent assignment that allowed me to take and pass the written part of general surgical boards in Heidelberg, Germany (where I also got to drive on the famous German Autobahn).

While in France, I treated several young soldiers who had sustained frost bite of the feet while stationed in Korea. This resulted in excessive sweating of the feet called hyperhidrosis. In addition, the arteries to the lower extremities went into spasm, or vasoconstriction, with impaired circulation and oftentimes, ulcerations. The end result was varying degrees of debilitation of significant degree, including feet rotting through boots.

The sympathetic nervous system (or autonomic or involuntary nervous system) is present throughout the body. As described above it is out of our control as compared with the voluntary nervous system such as walking, moving our eyes, speaking etc. This sympathetic nervous system has many functions, including stimulating our sweat glands to pour out fluid and our blood vessels to constrict. If the sympathetics to a lower extremity were blocked or removed that extremity would no longer sweat and the blood vessels would be relaxed with no compromised blood supply.

To demonstrate the presence or absence of sweating, a simple test may be used with iodine and starch. Sprinkling white starch powder on dry skin coated with iodine produces no change, but, if the surface is moist (such as sweating), the iodine would mix with the starch turning the latter blue.

We studied these afflicted soldiers. Lumbar sympathetic nerve injections using Novocain were administered resulting in temporary blockage of the nerves to the involved leg. The extremity became warm and dry. Before the block, the moist extremity that had been coated with iodine solution remained moist and with white starch powder added, the granules turned blue. Next, lumbar sympathetic block was done and the extremity dried up. The iodine solution was applied and allowed to dry. The starch powder then applied remained dry and white. With these satisfactory results, the patients underwent lumbar sympathectomy, or removal of these nerves to the involved leg. The results were excellent with elimination of a very morbid debilitating condition and restoration of these young adults to full duty.

I delivered a paper on the above at a military medical conference in Orleans, a suburb of Paris, which later appeared in the *Armed Forces Medical Journal, European Theatre, 1954.*

While in France I heard that a good friend from Syracuse, Dr. Al Falcone, was stationed with the U.S. Air Force in Europe, but I did not know where. One day I heard someone on the phone at our medical installation, talking with a Lieutenant Falcon in Bordeaux, France. It turned out to be my friend and we had many great talks. Al had not yet completed his general surgical training, let alone his plastic surgery, and therefore referred several burn cases requiring skin grafts. We still laugh about this.

At La Rochelle the chief surgeon of the area was Colonel Paul Milton. He was a portly, middle-aged fellow from Florida. It was understood that he practiced surgery there and recently re-entered the military during the Korean conflict as a "full bird." His work was strictly administrative, but it was obvious that he was a frustrated surgeon and he used to try to intimidate the younger surgeons. He did this with me but backed off when I indicated that his pressure was interfering with my work.

Interestingly, two years later I traveled from Denver to St, Louis, Missouri to take part in General Surgical Board Exams. These were oral. Much time was spent waiting outside the exam rooms with other examinees. In talking with a surgeon from Florida I asked if he knew Dr. Paul Milton. He laughed and said he knew him very well. He told me a story about Milton drinking heavily at a party and swallowing his denture, which led to an emergency esophagoscopy to remove the foreign body! If only I'd known this in La Rochelle!

Incidentally I passed the oral exam and became board certified in general surgery.

Chapter Five

THE DENVER EXPERIENCE

To my delight, my application for the thoracic surgical residency at National Jewish Hospital (NJH) was accepted and I was soon discharged from the medical corps in early 1955. While in France, I met a great fellow from Iowa City, Iowa, Dr. Jim Bauer. He was finishing up a final tour in the regular Army medical corps and we became very good friends. He arranged for me to spend six months on the surgical service of the VA hospital in Iowa City. It was a wonderful experience and nicely filled the six months between discharge and starting the chest residency. It introduced me to thoracic surgery, working under board certified thoracic surgeon Dr. Sam Walker. He was awfully good to me and prepared me well for the future.

While working in Iowa City, I traveled to Denver and briefly met Dr. John Grow, where he was operating at Children's Hospital. He was pleasant and cordial and I looked forward to my next assignment.

Arriving in Denver in June, 1955, I was very happy to see Chuck Demong after a hiatus of more than two years, although we had been communicating on occasion by mail.

He had been tremendously influential in my training during my surgical residency and I was eager to resume where we had left off. My dream was to eventually join Demong and Dr. John Grow in their thriving Denver practice.

I went to NJH, next and immediately noticed its motto on a huge sign in front of the hospital, "No one can enter who can pay and no one can pay to enter". I met Dr. Mauricio Goldberg from Argentina, who had worked as a fellow in chest surgery at NJH the past year. I was shocked when he informed me Dr. Grow had told him he would be the first-year resident in chest surgery and that I would be a fellow! I said nothing but immediately went to locate Dr. Grow. I was 32 years old, with two years of military medical experience, and many adult responsibilities. I confidently showed Dr. Grow the document confirming me as resident and told him that I fully expected to have that role. Without any outward emotion he backed down and accepted me as resident.

Perhaps that foretold my future in Denver. As events occurred over the next two years, I found Dr. Grow to be the most passive-aggressive individual that I have ever met before or since. Although I did not realize it immediately, it soon became apparent that my dream of working long term with him and Dr. Demong would never materialize.

To his credit, Dr. Grow allowed me to do both the surgery at NJH and much more of his private surgery than I ever imagined. Outwardly, we got along very well and never had a hot disagreement. But it was not the collegial environment I imagined before arriving. Charlie Demong proved to be a very different person than the one I knew in Syracuse. Dr. John Grow was in total charge and Demong was a shell of his former self.

Mauricio and I became very good friends and worked harmoniously together. It was always accepted that I was the resident and he was the fellow. (A few years later, after moving back to Syracuse, Mauricio visited me to ask if he could work with me. I kindly thanked him for his interest, but indicated that this was not possible and he returned to Baltimore, Maryland.)

It was a very tough, demanding residency at NJH. As the first-year and only resident I was extremely busy caring for patients before, during, and after surgery. I was on call 24-hours-a-day for the year, at a salary of $7,000.

These patients required a great deal of attention and care. There were many draining chest wounds. Diagnostic procedures as bronchography and bronchoscopy were required of all of the operative cases. The lung surgery was difficult on chronically ill patients with limited lung reserve and usually with disease in both lungs. Almost all of the chest surgery consisted of lung resections; the challenge was to conserve as much lung tissue as possible even though the retained lung had residual disease. Often times a modified thoracoplasty was done at the time of lung resection with excellent results and no space problems.

I was allowed to do well over 95 percent of the lung surgery myself and usually operated without attendings Grow or Demong. To put it mildly, it was a workout and no place for boys.

Near the end of my first year, I learned that the second year of preceptorship would no longer be recognized and accepted by the board of thoracic surgery for training and that a second year of residency would be required. A preceptorship consisted of working under a board certified chest surgeon on his/her private chest cases. The situation with Dr. Grow was excellent in that he had a tremendously busy private practice working in five hospitals, including a children's hospital. He was generous with his residents and allowed them to do much of the surgery. But this wasn't going to help me with the new change in requirements.

When I went to discuss this with Dr. Grow, his response was not surprising. He asked what I was going to do! He mentioned the possibility of my leaving Denver since I had passed my boards in general surgery. The implication was not to complete my chest training. He never once offered any assistance. Perhaps he was testing me or just wanted to see me squirm. In any case, I was ready. I calmly suggested that sending his cardiac surgical patients with restricted finances to NJH for surgery would create a second year residency and solve the problem. No further discussion ensued and with little fanfare this came to be. A two-year residency at NJH was approved by the Board of Thoracic Surgery.

This excellent training experience exposed me to many unique cases. J. W. was a 30-year old-male admitted to NJH with a history of repeated episodes of pneumonia in the right lung since five years of age. He had a draining wound in the right chest since the second of four operations performed between the ages five and nine to drain abscesses of the lung. Food particles had been noted in the large amounts of mucopurulent drainage.

In spite of this handicap, he had worked regularly as an auto mechanic. On examination, the patient was thin and appeared chronically ill. There was a defect in the right anterolateral chest wall beneath the axilla that measured 17cm in diameter. The ribs in this area had been resected. The floor of the defect contained numerous small bronchial fistulas. A bronchoscopic exam revealed a normal left bronchial tree, but there was granulation tissue and narrowing at the right intermediate bronchus. The bronchogram revealed marked contraction and severe bronchiectasis of all lobes of the right lung. On esophagoscopy, inflammation of the mucosa 34 cm from the upper incisors was noted. X-ray study of the esophagus failed to reveal a fistula but, barium particles were noted in the wound following this exam. Surgery was recommended and the attending, Dr. Demong, suspected a fistula or communication between the esophagus and the lung.

At surgery, there was complete obliteration of the plural space by dense adhesions. A pleuropneumonectomy was performed. There was a smooth elastic fistula connecting the esophagus to the right intermediate bronchus, which measured 7mm in length and 5mm in diameter. The fistulous tract was divided and the opening in the esophagus closed. The size of the remaining pleural space was reduced by a Bjork type thoracoplasty. The chest wall defect was closed after the debridement and a rubber tube brought out from the pleural space and connected to the water-seal drainage.

The patient was discharged three months later. His wounds were well-healed and he had no difficulty swallowing. Operating time: 7 hours; blood transfusion 4,500cc.

This condition is extremely rare. In 1945 Mullard reviewed the literature on this subject and was able to collect 30 cases of congenital tracheo-esophageal fistula and only three had been treated surgically. He added two cases of his own treated surgically.

In 1957, an article by Demong, Grow and G. Heitzman appeared in the *American Surgeon* and reported three cases of congenital tracheo-esophageal fistula and one case of broncho-esophageal fistula in their own personal experience in Denver. The broncho-esophageal fistula case is that of J. W.

Of the total of four cases successfully treated, they represented the fifth, sixth and seventh such cases reported in the world literature in 1957. (A note to medical students--One must always consider a congenital connection between the esophagus and lungs in cases of repeated lung infections, particularly where there is a draining chest wound with evidence of food material in the drainage.)

While this is an example of one of the most unique surgical cases I encountered, I treated many, many patients with tuberculosis. NJH was world renowned for the treatment of TB and people from all over the U.S.A and many foreign traveled to the hospital for treatment. This included Eskimo children from Alaska as well as those afflicted from the Hungarian Revolution in the 1950s.

Until the advent of anti-microbial treatment in the 1940s, there was only rest, diet, and collapse therapy. Most infections were pulmonary, although any organ is susceptible. The condition Addison's disease--involving the outer portion or cortex of the adrenal glands--was almost exclusively caused by this bacillus.

In instances of a cavity, sometimes a pneumothorax was administered--injecting air into the vacuum space between the chest wall and the lung. The cavities were almost always in the upper lung or lobe, and air installation or pneumothorax with its volume carefully controlled would result in that upper lobe collapsing and with it the cavity. It was postulated that the cavity would heal more readily if the wall collapsed on itself. Healing or arresting this disease was considered in terms of months and years and occupied a great deal of one's life.

A second and more definitive treatment was thoracoplasty. This meant removal of the upper ribs where the lung disease was present and allowed the soft tissue of the chest wall remaining to collapse on the underlying cavitated lung. This was done in stages of two to three ribs at a time, depending on the degree of lung involvement. Although this was effective treatment it was rather mutilating and deforming even on casual glance.

It should be stressed that drug failures were very common in the treatment of TB. In the 1950s, the antimicrobial Isoniazid was the treatment of choice and was extremely effective providing that the patient remained on it for at least two years. Unfortunately, many did not. Often, a patient felt so improved after a few weeks that the INH was discontinued. The organism is extremely slow growing when compared to a staff or strep and requires approximately two years for a curative result. Needless to say, many across the country and the world experienced this sensational improvement, only to have it short-lived by discontinuance of the drug and then experience drug resistance as a result.

My very best friend in Denver proved to be a patient, Ben Zeidman. As with most patients at NJH, Ben had a tubercle bacillus resistant to antimicrobial treatment with cavities in the lung. Surgical removal of a drug resistant lung was very dangerous because of the high complication rate. For several years before my arrival, surgery for these patients consisted of collapsing the cavity-containing lung. A popular method used had been plombage rather than the more complicated thoracoplasty, which required removal of several ribs and resulted in lung collapse. With plombage, an incision was made between the upper ribs at the site of the underlying lung cavity. With the cavity collapsed, plumbage materials (leucite balls, ivalon sponges or paraffin trimmed to the appropriate size) are placed between the chest wall and lung to maintain the cavity collapse. The rationale was that a cavity collapse on itself would heal. Frequently, irritation by the paraffin material resulted in infection and chronic drainage, usually containing tubercle bacilli. The drainage was chronic for years.

Ben was a New Yorker in his 50s who started and ran a successful appliance business. He came to the Mile High City with serious active TB. Several years before he had plombage performed by Dr. Grow and developed infection from the paraffin used with chronic draining sinus tract in the chest. This required daily dressings and considerable care. I took care of him for approximately two years and one of my biggest regrets in leaving Denver was departing from this fine man as he died after I left town.

It should be noted that the bacteriology lab at NJH was without peer. Its director was Gardner Middlebrook, PhD, recipient of the Louis Pasteur Award, and Pasteur is considered the Father of Bacteriology. His laboratory was extremely successful in culturing a tubercle bacillus from most patients and his methods of sensitivity to drugs were outstanding.

Chest surgery in the 1950s was in the pioneering stage. Cardiovascular surgery was in its infancy and there were few well-defined guidelines and techniques to follow. If one waited until reading about a new procedure in the surgical journals, he or she would not remain current, as the field progressed so rapidly. Dr. Grow was always current. He had a great network with other outstanding chest surgeons dating back to his days at Fitzsimmons Army Hospital and he was a wise politician. He frequently traveled to the active cardiac surgical centers all over North America and had first-hand familiarity with the latest methods.

He was a good looking fellow and could present himself in a charming manner. Moreover, he had terrific self confidence and backed this up by performing superbly in the operating room. I never saw him lose control in spite of any catastrophe encountered. He had large, powerful, hands and wore a size 8 ½ glove.

Dr. Grow instinctively knew how to operate and avoid difficulties. This was impossible all of the time in chest surgery because of the limitations of available technique. In spite of the problems at hand, with his steadiness and confidence he rarely ran into a situation beyond his control.

When I started in private practice and could not call on Dr. Grow to bail me out, I followed the lessons learned from him to remain calm and "not lose it." This almost always succeeded in taking care of the problem.

He once commented during my placement of a Hufnagel valve for aortic regurgitation, "George, you do better on your own," probably the nicest remark he ever gave me. I knew then I was ready to solo!

In spite of our differences and my disappointments with him personally, John Benson Grow helped me immensely to develop as a better surgeon and I am indebted to him for that.

There was a very strong bond between the patients at NJH and myself these two years. In June 1957, just before I left, we gathered together and they presented me with a gift of money they had collected among themselves. I was visibly shaken and expressed my gratitude for giving me something they had so little of.

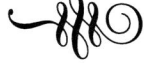

Chapter Six

THE MIRACLE PATIENT

One of the most amazing experiences in my professional life occurred at NJH in June 1957 near the completion of my thoracic surgery residency. In fact, it was the last heart operation I performed there.

The patient was a 10-year-old girl from Wilson, Kansas, Susan Kasper. She was an extremely bright, beautiful youngster with a congenital heart condition, secundum-type interatrial septal defect--an opening between the two reservoir chambers of the heart. This type of defect was amenable to repair using general body hypothermia—packing the body in ice to reduce body temperature to 30 degrees and reduce the tissues' need for blood. Ceasing total-body circulation can be safely done for at least 10 minutes. This was more time than required for this operation and similar cases had been successfully repaired here in recent months.

In fact, the very first successful open heart operation had been performed five years earlier by Dr. John Lewis at the University of Minnesota using hypothermia. His case was also an interatrial septal defect.

Dr. Grow's technique consisted of perfusing the

coronary arteries with warm, oxygenated blood during the cardiac bypass to nourish the coronaries.

Susan's surgery began normally. The defect was seen and repaired without difficulty. However, a tear had occurred in the opening into the right atrium and this required additional time to repair. Total interruption of the circulation was nine minutes, forty-five seconds, at which point the heart went into a ventricular fibrillation.

A few weeks earlier, while conducting experimental heart surgery on a dog, the animal's heart went into a similar ventricular fibrillation. After massaging the heart manually with my hand for 40 minutes, the heart began to beat normally again and the dog made a quick recovery.

I began massaging Susan's heart immediately. Eight electrical shocks were given, but fibrillation continued. Drugs were applied directly to the heart six times without result. We rewarmed her body by irrigating the chest lung cavities with warm saline while cardiac massage was continued to provide circulation to the brain and heart. After one hour of massage the temperature had risen to 32 degrees (normal is 37) and a normal heart rhythm spontaneously began.

We waited anxiously for her to come out of anesthesia, fearing brain damage that can result from prolonged interruption of the brain's oxygen supply (her total surgery time was one hour, 18 minutes). Miraculously, Susan awakened quickly and recognized her parents immediately. She recuperated uneventfully except for weakness of her lower extremities but had full recovery of her legs within a very brief time.

In September 1957, this operation was reported in *Time* magazine, in an article entitled "The Anxious Hour." Susan Kasper became the American Heart Association's "Valentine Girl" in 1958 and was greeted at ceremonies in Washington, DC, by President Eisenhower's wife, Mamie. She went on to become an outstanding scholar and was named Kansas "Outstanding Young Woman of the Year" in 1970. She graduated from the University of Kansas Medical School and became a pulmonologist, chief of internal medicine at the University of Kansas, and later, Scholar-in-Residence at the American Association of Medical Colleges in Washington, DC. We have communicated over the years and she has visited me in Syracuse. In one of my most cherished letters from patients, Susan wrote that the method used to save her inspired her to use aggressive treatment on her own patients during her career. She encouraged me to document my medical career, stressing the importance of sharing these experiences with current medical students.

As noted, in the 1950's I was trained in open heart surgery primarily with the use of hypothermia. Use of the heart-lung machine was in its infancy and there were many technicalities to understand and improve on than in hypothermia. The principle of the cooling technique is to slow down metabolism and reduce the requirement of oxygen. The most oxygen sensitive is nerve tissue, the brain and spinal cord. Without an adequate supply of oxygen beyond 2 to 4 minutes there is irreversible nerve tissue damage.

This is the limiting factor in using hypothermia in heart surgery rather than the heart or other organs that tolerate lack of oxygenated blood for periods of ten minutes or longer without problems at temperatures of 30 degrees C rectally.

Hibernating animals tolerate marked reduction of oxygen requirement in cold months without incident. Hibernation undoubtedly would have been studied in greater depth had not the heart-lung machine been developed so rapidly.

It is interesting to speculate on the need of the heart-lung machine if the hibernating phenomenon were successfully studied and solved. To apply the success of hibernation to humans is very interesting to speculate on. Would the heart-lung machine ever been necessary? Cooling methods used in association with the heart-lung machine have been employed successfully for many years in complex cardiac surgery.

Currently cooling methods have been used successfully in patients with sudden ischemia of the brain with severe heart attacks with the rationale of cooling the brain to reduce oxygen demand due to diminished blood supply and thus prevent permanent brain damage.

Hypothermia is a relatively simple technique with very rewarding results providing the temperatures are well controlled at 30 degrees C rectally and never below to prevent refractory cardiac arrhythmias.

There are more and more reports of success with severe heart attacks and cardiac arrest with associated cerebral anoxia.

In October 2010 at Upstate University Hospital, Syracuse, hypothermia was used on a 34 year-old male who suffered a massive heart attack to prevent brain damage. There was complete recovery.

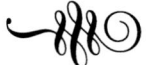

Chapter Seven

RETURNING TO MY ROOTS

Although I had learned a tremendous amount from Dr. Grow, I clearly realized that that my dream of being welcomed into private practice with him and Dr. Demong was not meant to be. There were other options. Dr. Al Kukral, a previous resident at NJH about three years my senior invited me to join him in private practice. He was very successful but practiced largely general surgery. There would be little to no heart surgery and not much thoracic. I had a similar offer at a clinic in Colorado Springs.

I could see no point in having done these last two years of training only to practice general surgery, particularly since I enjoyed chest surgery so much more. I decided to go home after being away five years to develop a practice in Syracuse.

My parents and Jim were elated.

I contacted the director of surgery at Upstate Medical Center. He felt I did not have enough laboratory background to be a full time thoracic surgeon in his department but did offer a stipend to work in the laboratory with a heart-lung machine under a full-time general surgeon. I did this along with giving talks to the surgical staff on hypothermia and open heart surgery. Many people seemed intrigued but nothing materialized.

My brother had returned to Syracuse two years earlier. Along with his private practice, he was Medical Director at St. Joseph's Hospital for a short time. Jim. had a lovely office in the State Tower Building downtown, which was easily accessible to St. Joe's. He graciously shared this with me for many months free of rent, and we remained together in this office with classmate Carl Austin, an internist, until 1980. My hero came through again.

Soon the surgical director at Upstate informed me that a full-time chest surgeon was joining his department. I had already entertained thoughts of trying to duplicate what John Grow did in Denver, a much larger city of over one million. As soon as Grow entered private practice, facilities at Children's Hospital were arranged for open heart surgery with hypothermia, along with closed heart operations in several hospitals. Soon he was the busiest, most respected, and successful heart surgeon in the area, much more so than his peers at the academic Colorado Medical Center. Grow's history was known by the surgical director at Upstate through a close friend in Denver and he advised me "not to try doing in Syracuse what was done in Denver."

I said nothing and resigned from the department of

surgery at Upstate. I never spoke with him again.

I had already contacted Dr. Carl Geiger, chief of anesthesia at St. Joseph's Hospital, about starting an open heart surgery program there. Carl was interested and advised me to talk with the Delmonicos. Dr. Ernie Delmonico, Sr. was in his early sixties and a very powerful general surgeon who had been formally chief for many years. His son Ernie, Jr. was a thoracic surgeon, four years my senior. He had excellent thoracic training at the Overholt Clinic in Boston, including a six months in Philadelphia with the famous Dr. Charles Bailey. Ernie was very busy with closed heart surgery, particularly mitral valve procedures. He had no training in open heart surgery.

Both Delmonicos were very receptive to this idea. Ernie, Jr. and I met with the hospital administrator, Sister Wilhelmina, Monsignor Joseph Toomey, who was very active in hospital activities, and well-known Syracuse banker Tom Higgins. All were extremely interested in bringing open heart surgery to St. Joseph's and Central New York.

In order to proceed further, we needed someone to do the heart catheterizations and other studies that diagnose the conditions amenable to surgical correction under direct vision. With the consent of Sister Wilhelmina, I contacted Dr. Goffredo Gensini, whom I knew from Denver. He had recently arrived in Denver from Italy, and trained with well-known Denver cardiologist Gil Blount in heart catheterization and other associated laboratory studies. Dr. Gensini had become chief of the cardio-respiratory lab at NJH shortly before I left Denver.

Initially, Dr. Gensini and a technician flew from Denver to Syracuse once a month on weekends. They both lived in my home and a group of children were studied under makeshift conditions in the radiology department at St. Joseph's. Dr. Delmonico and I funded their expenses.

My own private practice grew immediately at St. Joseph's, where many of my friends practiced. My first chest operation was on D.W. She had an asymptomatic mass picked up on a routine chest x-ray taken at the State Fair. The mass was located in the mediastinum, an area occupied by the heart, esophagus, and other structures. The mass proved to be a benign dermoid cyst. It was excised and her recovery was excellent.

D. had been referred by Dr. Marshal Fulmer. Dr. Fulmer's office was immediately adjacent to the street I grew up on in East Syracuse. Interestingly, this short street of two blocks housed seven M.D.s who had lived or were raised there over two generations: Dr. Tom Snyder and his father Mat, both general practitioners in town; Martin Coyne, Blaine Amidon, Ray Seagfried (our family doctor), Jim and myself. I believe this is a rare statistic in a railroad town of 5,000 people.

Within a short time, a number of patients in need of open heart surgery were found. Sister Wilhelmina and Monsignor Toomey flew to Denver to interview Dr. Gensini further before offering him the position of Director of the cardiopulmonary lab. He accepted the position and became director of the Msgr. Toomey Cardiopulmonary Laboratory and Research Department.

Dr. Gensini moved to Syracuse with his wife Ena, daughter Gioia, and Ena's parents. They purchased a house across the street in my neighborhood. Our relationship was very cordial and we socialized but, they were rather private.

Dr. Gensini was personable and energetic. He performed very well in the hospital and was very pleasant to work with. Soon, more and more cardiac adult cases were referred for study, largely with rheumatic mitral and aortic valve problems; those with coronary artery disease followed. Cardiologist Asher Black showed great interest in coronary artery disease and initially many of the patients studied were referred by him.

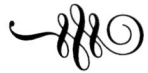

Chapter Eight

BRINGING OPEN HEART SURGERY TO SYRACUSE

The terms closed heart and open heart surgery should be further defined. Closed heart surgery refers to operations that are performed on a normal beating heart, frequently penetrating one or more chambers digitally and/or with a cutting or dilating instrument. These procedures are usually to open a narrowed valve, congenital or acquired, particularly the mitral, aortic, or pulmonic. The most frequent heart surgeries had been performed on the mitral valve, as statistically this was the most affected by rheumatic fever with resulting narrowing. In my opinion--and one shared by most of my fellow heart surgeons--Dr. Charles Bailey was the greatest contributor to the development of closed heart surgery. He was brilliant, eccentric, determined and capable.

While closed heart surgery involving the mitral valve had been done in the 1920s with rare success, Bailey dramatically popularized closed methods with acceptable results. In the 1950s he went on to train hundreds of residents, including Ernie Delmonico, Jr. He was an extremely capable technician and felt that most mitral valve stenosis required a cutting knife rather than the finger alone, and his residents were trained accordingly. This was not the case in most training centers, including my own. I learned how to use these knives from Ernie.

In spite of helping thousands of patients through a closed method, most heart problems required a more precise deliberate approach, namely open heart surgery. With the latter, one or more heart chambers were opened and the defect(s) visualized and corrected. This includes holes between chambers, and narrowed valves, with and without regurgitation. Many times the valves are so diseased they must be replaced.

Hypothermia had been studied for many years and it was known to slow metabolism. In the 1950s, several investigators in Toronto, Minneapolis and Denver studied its application to heart surgery. It was learned that with rectal temperature of 30 Celsius (normal is 37 C), circulation could be stopped for at least 10 minutes with survival. At 37 C, the brain and nervous system would be permanently damaged after three minutes with no circulation.

At the time, there were a number of congenital heart defects that could be corrected in 10 minutes at 30 C. In 1952, Dr. John Lewis, reported the first successful open heart surgery in history by repairing an interatrial-septal defect, secundum type, using hypothermia. This led to hundreds of cases successfully operated with the cooling technique. For the most part, relatively simple congenital heart defects could be repaired because of the time limitation required to correct more complicated problems where the bypass would be necessary. To do these procedures the heart must be arrested and replaced by an artificial heart-lung machine.

Very early in the 1950s, the Minnesota group used a cross circulation technique for children's surgery where an adult with the same blood type, frequently a parent, would act as a heart-lung machine because his/her circulation would be connected to the patient's. This posed many risks and limitations and was shortly discontinued.

Many brilliant investigators were involved in developing an artificial heart-lung machine. In 1953, Philadelphia cardiac surgeon Dr. John Gibbons, perfected a machine and successfully used it on a young girl with an interatrial-septal defect. This was the first successful open heart operation using a heart-lung machine. Thereafter, more and more successes were reported with other machines. The Mayo Clinic further perfected his model and it became known as the Mayo-Gibbons heart-lung.

Without reservation, the key to starting an open heart program at St. Joseph's Hospital was Sister Wilhelmina. I am forever grateful to this fine, quiet, and bright woman for encouraging us to proceed with this project. She had great vision. This open heart program would not have succeeded at this hospital but for her. Her presence at this time was an absolute necessity.

State approval of the heart program in each hospital was required and this necessitated hands-on affirmation by the state for open cardiovascular procedures. Officials came and scrutinized our Msgr. Toomey cardiopulmonary lab. In 1958 two heart surgeons and professors, Dr. James Mahoney, from Strong Memorial Hospital in Rochester, and Dr. Ralph Alley from Albany Medical Center, visited and observed an open heart procedure on separate occasions. Everything went well. In fact Dr. Mahoney said that he had never before seen a case of isolated infundibular pulmonic stenosis, which we performed on his day of observation. After many months of requests and preparation for all of this we were finally approved. Actually state approval was more of a moral than a financial victory and demonstrated that we were a qualified recognized state entity.

On November 12, 1958, after numerous rehearsals of the procedure with dogs as subjects, eight-year-old Sharon Melfi underwent the first open heart surgery in Syracuse at St. Joseph's Hospital under hyperthermia. With her body temperature lowered to 30 C, we were able to clamp off circulation to her heart, allowing the heart to be opened to repair the valve that controls blood flow for the heart to the artery leading to the lung—in technical terms, a valvulotomy was carried out under direct vision for a tight pulmonic stenosis and obstruction of the flow of blood from the heart into the lungs.

Sharon's heart was open for about five minutes for the procedure. As soon as the heart was closed, warm water was circulated through a blanket to rewarm her body. Once her body reached normal temperature, about two hours later, she began a rapid recovery. Her postoperative course was very satisfactory. Sharon went on to become a nurse and then marry and have three children.

The next month, 10-year-old Paula O'Connell underwent closure of a defect measuring the size of a fifty-cent piece between the walls of the upper chambers of the heart, an interatrial septal defect, secundum type. Just five years earlier, she would have been doomed. Hypothermia with adjunct measures was used again successfully. Both of these surgeries were front-page news in the Syracuse newspapers.

When the open heart surgical program was initiated at St. Joseph's, there was no surgical insurance coverage, including that for the indigent. Concerning the private health insurance companies, we had a battle and many discussions and debates ensued. After some months of wrangling with the president of Blue Cross/Blue Shield, approval for insurance coverage was granted. In time all private insurances covered, in various percentages, doctor and hospital bills for open heart operations.

Shortly after the first open heart procedures in 1958 Sister Wilhelmina was taking steps to start the first intensive care unit in CNY at St. Joseph's. This was on floor 3-R, a general surgical unit. It was headed by a recent St. Joseph's graduate, Patricia O'Neil. She selected new graduates, Stella Sroka and Mary Pat Doran and these formed an outstanding team. The unit rapidly grew from 8 beds in 2 rooms. In time Patricia married resident anesthesiologist Dr. Tom Donnelly and they moved to Auburn, New York. Mary Pat married Peter Coleman, owner of the famous Irish Pub on Tipperary Hill on the west side and retired. Stella grew with the hospital, becoming director of the expanding ICU. She then took other responsible nursing duties and became one of the true nursing greats. She had all of the ingredients to become an outstanding physician.

Within the open heart program, rapid progress continued and many unsung heroes and heroines were involved. Sister Laurine stood out. She was a young nurse who had recently come to Syracuse from her native Hawaii. She was selected by Sister Wilhelmina to be closely allied with the heart surgeons and was most helpful and supportive in multiple roles. She had great enthusiasm and drive and was always positive. A major contribution was to operate the heart-lung machine, and often Sister Laurine would work the eight-hour ICU shift after operating the heart-lung.

With administrator Sister Wilhelmina in charge, heart surgery and work in the lab flourished. While in Denver, Gensini's forte had been in the laboratory diagnosing congenital heart problems. With the friendship of Mason Sones in Cleveland, he became very proficient in the lab study of acquired heart disease, particularly of the coronaries, and he contributed to the medical literature with the Gensini Catheter. He soon was assisted by Dr. Peter Huntington, a formally trained clinical board-certified cardiologist who joined to acquire cardiac catheterization and associated techniques.

Drs. Paulo Essente and Alex Giambartolomei arrived from Italy to work in the lab. They were industrious, bright, and capable physicians. With more study, Alex went on to become a board-certified cardiologist. Paulo remained in the laboratory, and was very capable and comfortable to work with. Along with Peter, they were great compliments as assistant directors in the department.

I would be remiss if Miss Ann Kelly was omitted mention. She was a delightful, bright, good natured R.N. graduate from St. Joseph's who had an intense interest in the lab. She started there in its infancy and remained working there for many years. She, too, was instrumental in the development of the cardiopulmonary laboratory.

The Forrester heart-lung machine was purchased by the hospital in 1961. Use of a heart-lung allowed much longer operating time and thus the ability to perform more complicated surgery, both congenital as well as acquired, such as valve replacements. We went directly to the animal lab and perfected procedures before its use on humans. George More, trained in machinery repair and maintenance, became a close associate of Sister Laurine and was extremely dependable and supportive in operating and servicing all of the equipment. Shortly thereafter, the hospital purchased the Mayo-Gibbon heart lung, considered to be the finest available.

Sister Wilhelmina sent Sister Laurine to the Mayo Clinic, Rochester, Minnesota to be instructed in its use. This was a tremendous experience and was extremely valuable to everyone concerned. In a short time all open heart surgery was done with the heart-lung, with and without hypothermia, and there was no longer a time limit to perform these operations safely. Nevertheless, hypothermia alone had an essential role in early open heart procedures at St. Joseph's Hospital and many lives were saved before the heart-lung was perfected.

Dr. Delmonico and I paid for George More's trip to Mayos where he too learned the mechanics and details in running the Mayo-Gibbons machine.

Chapter Nine

A NEW ERA IN HEART SURGERY

With the acquisition of the heart-lung machine, the bulk of open heart surgery shifted to adults and to more complicated surgical procedures. These included opening narrowed and or leaking valves and replacing them.

In 1959, Dr. Mason Sones at the Cleveland Clinic introduced and perfected coronary arteriography, using dye to outline the coronary arteries to detect obstructions. Dr. Gensini became a close friend and soon brought this technique to St. Joseph's. Consequently, a large number of cases were studied for coronary disease, and beginning in 1964, the Vineberg operation for angina was started at St. Joseph's.

Coronary Artery Disease and Angina

The surgical treatment of coronary artery disease had been attempted for several decades. Prior to the use of the heart-lung machine and coronary bypass its treatment has had many limitations. In the 1940s and 50s cardiac surgeon Claude Beck introduced the use of talc poudrage. This consisted of abrading the heart surface and applying talc powder, which is an irritant. All patients were studied preoperatively with coronary arteriograms and significant coronary arteriosclerosis with narrowing was demonstrated. One patient, J.R, was 21 years post-procedure when seen for the last time and doing very well.

In 1946, Arthur Vineberg, a Montreal surgeon in private practice, reported a method of revascularizing the heart with benefit. He initially perfected his procedure in the laboratory. His method of improving the circulation consisted of implanting a bleeding artery into a tunnel created in the wall of the cardiac muscle shown to be lacking a satisfactory blood supply. It required six to eight weeks for connections (collaterals) between the coronary arteries and the newly introduced artery to develop. This was not widely accepted as it could not be proven beneficial in humans until 1959 when Dr. Sones introduced selective coronary arteriography (injecting dye into the heart vessels and taking moving picture x-rays). He demonstrated collaterals in his patients between the internal mammary and coronary arteries.

At St. Joseph's, we had considerable experience with this procedure with a very low mortality rate and surprisingly good results. Using the Vineberg method, between 1964 and 1970, 47 patients underwent single- or double-internal mammary artery implants at St Joseph's Hospital. The operative mortality was 6.4 percent and 72 percent were angina free or unproved; 79 percent of the implants were patent and functioning.

A most unusual and satisfying case is that of S.B. He had experienced his first heart attack at age 32. Repeated obstruction occurred with associated chest pain and very limited physical activity. A coronary arteriogram (special x-rays that outline the coronary arteries of the heart using dye) at St. Joe's demonstrated satisfactory filling of the right coronary but near total obstructions of the two major left coronaries. A left Vineberg was done in 1964 when he was 36. At surgery, several old infarcts (healed areas of dead heart tissue) were present and examination was limited due to cardiac irritability. Two post-op arteriograms demonstrated excellent collaterals from the implant.

Mr. B. did well until some years later when angina recurred and progressed. A repeat coronary arteriogram showed complete occlusion of the right coronary. A right implant was done on in 1969 with good recovery. When last seen six-months-later, he had an excellent clinical result. He was actually living on his two implants, and admittedly, this was very gratifying to me.

Our St. Joseph's experience with the Vinebergs was nicely summarized in an article co-written by myself with Drs. Huntington, Gensini, and Delmonico, published in the *New York State Medical Journal* in 1972.

Aorto Coronary Bypass

In 1964, Michael DeBakey performed the first successful aorto-coronary bypass using an autogenous saphenous vein, with confirmation of the functioning graft by arteriogram seven years later. During that same period of time, in 1967, Rene Favalaro at the Cleveland Clinic perfected a saphenous aorto-coronary bypass and reported on 100 patients operated. These were the first reported cases of direct bypass of the blocked coronary arteries.

These surgeries initially were done using veins, and later, arteries. Many times the veins occluded, which was attributed to the high pressure on the vein wall. For that reason arteries are now used whenever possible.

In 1970, I performed the first aorta-coronary saphenous vein bypass graft (bypassing an obstructed coronary artery with a vein taken from the leg and interposed between the aorta and coronary beyond the obstruction) in Syracuse at St. Joseph's Hospital on 56-year-old C. K., for severe right coronary obstruction. He did extremely well until 1983, when angina recurred. A coronary arteriogram showed excellent function of the bypass done 13 years before. The recent angina was proven due to obstructive left coronary disease. Mr. K. died postoperatively at the age of 69.

Giant Coronary Artery Aneurysm With Fistulas

Giant coronary artery aneurysms with fistulas are rare. From July, 1963, to 2007, J.F. Howell, M.D., and Albert Raizner, M.D., of Methodist DeBakey Heart and Vascular Center, in Houston Texas, performed 30,000 cardiac or vascular operations. Among these, only three patients had giant coronary artery aneurysms with fistulas and these underwent surgical correction.

In my experience from 1958-1972 there were two such cases.

M. H., a 54-year-old woman with an enlarged heart for 15 years was under the care of Dr. Paul Maglione for three years and hospitalized in 1964 for heart failure. She improved on digitalis and a low-salt diet. A heart catheterization (diagnostic test with introduction of a catheter into the heart chambers to determine pressures in the or associated abnormal connections) in the summer of 1964 showed a patent ductus arteriosis (congenital connection between pulmonary artery and aorta normally sealing off spontaneously shortly after birth). During surgical consultation, this diagnosis was questioned because of the location of the machinery murmur.

Repeat catheterization disclosed a fistula arising from the left coronary artery and entering the superior vena cava-right atrium area. The size of the fistula was enormous.

Surgery was recommended and accepted.

The operative findings disclosed an enormous aneurysmal sac extending from the left main coronary artery over the dorsal aspect of the heart, namely over the left atrium dorsal to the right pulmonary artery and emptying into the junction of the superior vena cava and right atrium in its lateral aspect. The aneurysm measured up to 5 cm and greatest diameter and calcium deposits were scattered throughout its length.

Using the Mayo-Gibbon Heart-Lung via a sternal split and hypothermia, the sac was entered with the ascending aorta clamped. The origin of the fistula was closed with interrupted sutures, followed by closure of the sac. The postoperative course was uneventful.

R. D. was first studied at St. Joseph's at age 10 and a heart catheterization revealed increased oxygen saturation in the right ventricle. The right heart pressures were normal and it was felt he had a ventricular-septal defect and required no treatment at that time. Over the ensuing years he felt well but, but was becoming more fatigued. He was referred to me by his primary physician, Dr. Tom Bishop of Minoa, at age 20.

Repeat heart catheterization, left and right, was performed at St. Joseph's and a huge right coronary artery to right ventricular fistula was demonstrated. The pressure studies of the left and right heart chambers were normal. There was an estimated two-to- one ratio of right ventricular flow as compared with the left. Surgical correction was recommended by the cardiac review board because of the incidence of endocarditis, aneurysmal blow-out, and cardiac failure.

On October 30, 1968, with heart-lung standby, a sternotomy incision was made and the findings confirmed the above. A huge right tortuous coronary artery became aneurysmal 2 cm-in-diameter as it entered the right ventricle near the posterior descending artery supplied by the left coronary. The right coronary artery was temporarily occluded and the aneurysmal enlargement emptied and the previously palpated thrill at this point disappeared. Here the right coronary was ligated and doubly transfixed.

The patient's operative and postoperative course was excellent and he thrived thereafter. In January, 1974, sternal wires were removed because of foreign body granulomata. When last seen the next month, five-and-a-half years post-op, it was felt he was in excellent condition and had a normal cardiovascular system.

Ventricular Aneurysm

According to *Bailey's Surgery of the Heart*: "Ventricular aneurysm may be defined as a relatively localized outpouching of the wall of a cardiac ventricle (pump) due to disease. This causes cardiac over work and enlargement and should be eliminated from the circulation by excision whenever possible. This is usually the result of gradual replacement of necrotic heart muscle by scar tissue following infarction (muscle death) due to coronary occlusion (obstruction). The healing results in a fibrous scar. On cut surface the wall of the ventricle is markedly thinned. If the area of infarction is enlarged it may begin to bulge outwardly with each contraction and will gradually become larger. The presence of this non-functioning pouch reduces the efficiency of the ventricular contractions with loss of cardiac reserve and eventual heart failure. Clots or thrombi develop on the inner surface of 50 percent of aneurysms and may break off and travel to various areas of the body, including the brain with resultant strokes. Congestive heart failure occurs in 70 percent and was the main cause of death in 41 percent. Thromboembolic phenomena were observed in 51.9 percent. These statistics are in marked contrast to 90 percent survival of infarction or rehabilitation in 85 percent of the surviving patients in the absence of aneurysm formation."

The first successful surgical treatment of a ventricular aneurysm in the human by excision was reported by Bailey in April, 1954, at the Hahnemann Hospital, in Philadelphia, conducted as a closed-heart procedure. This was in a 56-year-old-male whose initial myocardial infarction occurred in January 1953. The base of the aneurysm was clamped at its cephalad (toward head) 2/3 and the base closed with a continuous silk suture followed with interrupted mattress silk sutures. Following removal of the clamp the cut edges were approximated with continuous silk.

His postoperative course was excellent. He was able to climb two flights of stairs whereas he was unable to walk more than a few yards on the level preoperatively. This great benefit persisted when he was last seen one year after surgery.

At St. Joseph's Hospital, we treated eight patients (seven males and one female) with ventricular aneurysms between 1967 and 1971.

The most famous is Joe Palmieri, the only long-term statistic, who is alive and well at age 83 as of this writing in 2010.

The men in Joe's family had a terrible history of heart disease. His grandfather, father, two uncles, and two cousins all died of heart attacks. Joe had two heart attacks within 30 days of each other at age 34. While in the hospital recuperating, he complained of a "double" heartbeat. X-rays were ordered and Joe was told he had a "bubble" on the upper section of the heart, close to the aorta.

Although he endured some physical limitations, Joe lived a mostly normal life for the next six years. One day, at lunch with his cousin, Dr. Paul Maglione, his cousin listened to his heart with a stethoscope. Not liking what he heard, he booked Joe an appointment with Dr. Gensini for the following day. A catheterization revealed a 7cm. aneurysm in danger of bursting at any time. The bulge was engorged with thrombus; a stroke was imminent.

Joe was referred to me for surgery, which was scheduled for June 4, 1969. The aneurysm was carefully removed and the left ventricular chamber lavaged with saline to remove any possible thrombus remnants. The opening in the ventricle was then closed with mattress suture of #00 silk. Before the complete closure of the ventricular chamber, all air was removed by ventilating the lung. The aortic clamp was left on for about 20 minutes. When the clamp was removed, ventricular fibrillations ensued. This is a lethal irregular heart rate (arrhythmia). Paddles were applied directly to the left ventricle, one shock restored this to a normal beat.

Joe remained hospitalized for 30 days. Of that experience, he writes, "A few days later, I sensed that my heart began playing in perfect harmony. Every beat was a musical note of an Italian opera that ended, not with sorrow, but with overwhelming joy and exhilaration. I was 'flying' without the pain pills!"

After three weeks additional rehab at home, Joe returned to work with no physical restrictions except for running.

A few years later, after having moved to the Balitmore area, Joe experienced a tightening of the chest and called for an ambulance. He was admitted to the hospital and his physician determined a possible heart attack was near. Over the next five days, a number of heart tests were conducted. He was then released on the condition he return for a follow up the next week.

He continued to see the heart doctor for the next 25 years without event. If his heart felt uncomfortable, he'd go to the hospital as a precaution. In recent years, his heart developed atrial fibrillation. As he approached 80, his cardiologist recommended a pacemaker, which was installed in 2007.

While I have been unable to verify the fact through any professional organization, I strongly believe Joe may be the longest living patient from such a procedure, or at least the longest living to require no further open heart procedures.

We treated two male patients for ventricular aneurysm who were even younger and were operated on at ages 31 and 34. One had his first heart attack at age 28.

Of the eight cases, there were two deaths. A 44-year-old male had extensive coronary artery disease and marked destruction of the left ventricle. In retrospect, a heart transplant was necessary but not available at the time. The other, a 54-year-old man, died suddenly nine days after surgery of a cardiac arrythmia.

Today, the general age group undergoing left ventricular aneurysmectomy is considerably older, in the late fifties and beyond, Mortality is in the 2 percent range and surgery is done in conjunction with coronary bypass.

The world famous heart surgeon, Dr. Denton Cooley, of Houston, Texas, reported very early results of surgical excision of ventricular aneurysms in 1959, 10 years before the Joe Palmieri operation. His results were excellent in 10 patients, all operated on in 1958; all but two survived. These patients were in their forties and fifties. The two deaths were older. All had extensive coronary artery disease and this era preceded coronary artery bypass as did our series.

Takotsubo is left ventricular apical ballooning (LVAB) characterized by intermittent severe weakness of the apex of the heart muscle despite the presence of apparently normal coronary arteries. The typical case is one of a post menopausal woman with sudden chest pain, severe myocardial dysfunction and EKG changes consistent with a classic heart attack. In contrast early after the onset angiography shows no coronary obstruction.

This is also termed "broken heart" or stress cardiomyopathy as it is usually preceded by physical or emotional stress. Pulmonary edema may occur with a 2%

mortality. However, most patients recover spontaneously within one month with no irreversible heart damage. The prognosis is good and there is a 10% recurrence.

Japanese physicians originally described LVAB and thought the ballooning resembled an octopus trap (takotsubo). It is increasingly encountered in the U.S.A and Europe. With those diagnosed with a heart attack 2% of males and 12% of women may have LVAB. Physicians must be familiar with the condition and its treatment as anticoagulants and agents usually used for heart attacks may be contraindicated.

The mechanism involved is poorly understood. Paolo Angelini MD, cardiologist at the Texas Heart Institute, Houston, Texas has provided new insights. He found that acetylcholine provoked typical symptoms and EKG changes with extreme spasm of the coronary arteries. Intracoronary nitroglycerine resolved the symptoms, spasm and ballooning.

Dr. Angelini reports evidence that LVAB is due to severe multi vessel spasm in those with a variable degree of endothelial dysfunction and who are exposed to various stressors. In some cases large amounts of catecholamines (usually epinephrine) are released into the blood stream and may induce a temporary stunned state.

In addition, certain similarities exist between LVAB and Prinzmetal angina. In the latter a spasm occurs in a single coronary artery but does not last long enough to cause myorcardial stunning. In both conditions recurrence may be better prevented by calcium antagonists and nitrates than by other cardiovascular agents. Some researchers believe that LVAB is part of a group of related clinical entities that have a common pathophysiology. This concept awaits further testing.

The First Pacemaker in Syracuse

In 1963, I visited Denver for a surgical meeting. Dr. Adrian Kantrowitz, from Brooklyn, New York, known in the literature as a thoracic surgeon with great interest in research of the heart, presented for the very first time a new innovation--a pacemaker for heart block. Patients with this malady lost consciousness due to an extremely low heart rate and some never awakened. A rate of 50 beats per minute is invariably too low to sustain an adequate brain circulation even in superbly trained athletes.

The pacemaker at the meeting was manufactured by General Electric and well researched. The presentation drew considerable attention; it was the "pearl" of the meeting.

On returning home, I told my brother Jim about the pacemaker and within a week Drs. Carhart and Daley referred a patient with a heart block. On May 3, 1963, Dr. Delmonico and I implanted the first pacemaker in Syracuse at St. Joseph's.

The surgery was done through a left anterior chest

incision. The two electrodes were sutured to the left ventricle and a large battery, four inches in diameter, was placed using an incision in the left upper abdomen.

The battery was set at a rate of 70 stimuli per minute and guaranteed this heart rate.

Pacemaker technology has improved enormously. Soon the battery was reduced in size to 2 inches by ½ inch and placed in a very small incision under the skin below the left collar bone. The attached wires were introduced through a vein in the neck and placed within a chamber of the heart, the right atrium, to stimulate the conduction system controlling the heart rate. Over the decades it is gratifying to witness the improvements made in this field. The pacemakers are much smaller now and have amazing capabilities, including defibrillation of the heart when necessary.

As time went on more companies entered into this field and General Electric withdrew from the market. Medtronic, Cordis and Intermedics are commonly used with excellent results.

Tumors of the Heart

Tumors of the heart are rare. Primary tumors are those originating in the heart. Secondary are those whose origin is elsewhere. Secondary tumors are 20 to 40 times more common.

Of the primary tumors the ratio of benign to malignant is 16 to 1. Myxomas are benign and the most common. Seventy-five percent develop in the left atrium, 25 percent in the right. They usually grow in the septum or partition between the atria. As they grow, they project downward and often partially block the mitral valve, giving a ball-valve effect, and simulate intermittent mitral stenosis (narrowing) with shortness of breath. Change in position, from sitting to lying down for example, can change the tumor-valve relationship and relieve the symptoms. Prior to open heart surgery, attempts to remove these tumors were unsuccessful.

We treated two cases with excellent results.

E.D. was a 43-year-old-married female with a history of shortness of breath relieved by leaning forward. This was suggestive of a ball-valve obstruction of the mitral, such as myxoma.

During heart catheterization, she experienced a right hemiplegia, or stroke, and the procedure was not completed. With anticoagulation(blood thinners) and physiotherapy she improved markedly. A more complete heart evaluation was then done and a normal mitral valve found with slight regurgitation. The left atrium was not well-filled with dye, suggesting a ball- valve mechanism originating in this chamber. Open heart surgery was advised.

A vigorous pre-op treatment was carried out, resulting

in a 20-pound weight loss. On July 2, 1963, with heart-lung bypass, a 6-7 cm-in-diameter tumor arising from the interatrial septum was found and removed. The pathology report was myxoma and her postoperative course was uneventful thereafter. Possibly the right hemiplegia (stroke) was secondary to a portion of the tumor breaking off and traveling to the brain via the bloodstream.

The second patient, J. D., was a 52-year-old female referred by internist Dr. Tom Murphy in early December, 1971, for heart catheterization. She had a history of bouts of palpitation and four episodes of fainting over eight years. Heart catheterization was consistent with a tumor of the left atrium adjacent to the septum. Further history revealed an inability to lie on her left side.

Surgery was recommended by the cardiac review board. On December 29 1971, on cardiac bypass, the left atrium was entered via a right atriotomy and then opening the interatrial septum. A tumor 5 cm-in-diameter with a stalk 1.5 cm-in-diameter was found and excised from the septum.

Pathological report was myxoma. Postoperatively, her course was uneventful. Possibly her inability to lie on her left side was due to the tumor projecting into the mitral valve intermittently.

Subaortic Stenosis

Although common in canines, subaortic stenosis is relatively rare in humans. The congenital condition is an anatomic obstruction to egress of blood across the left ventricular outflow tract. The specific treatment is removal of the diaphragm without damaging important adjacent structures.

My personal cardiologist, who has had an extremely busy practice for approximately 20 years has seen only two cases. From 1958 to 1972 at St. Joseph's Hospital there was only one case.

Our patient, J. S., was 45 years old when she underwent heart surgery for subaortic valvular stenosis of the membranous type. (Others may be muscular in nature.) She had a heart murmur since childhood and a bout of subacute bacterial endocarditis at age 25. At 40, she developed heart failure and required digitalization and diuretics. A heart catheterization two-months earlier showed a marked obstruction one centimeter below a normal aortic valve with a pressure gradient of 120 mm Hg (LV inflow 185/ 22 LV outflow 65/28).

At open heart surgery through an incision in the ascending aorta, the aortic valve cusps were separated to reveal a fibrous diaphragm obstructing the outflow of the left ventricle. It measured 3 mm in thickness with a tiny aperture 4 mm in diameter. It was located 1 cm below the aortic valve.

This diaphragm was also attached to the aortic and mitral valves and ventricular septum. This was meticulously excised.

The patient's postoperative course was uneventful. When seen over three years later, she was totally asymptomatic. She had an excellent result. Fortunately this defect was very well localized without additional abnormalities.

"Without (surgery), he wouldn't have lived very long. People don't live this long after an operation. He's as sharp as a tack. It may be some kind of record, I don't know".

- *Heitzman on Joe Palmieri*

   Truly a heartfelt reunion – Monday, June 2, 2008.

   The Ithaca Journal

"Here I am, a little old man that he operated on. And when I saw him, geez, I just hugged him. Before I left, I kind of choked up a little bit".

- *Joe Palmieri*

   To Touch Hearts – Monday, June 16, 2008.

   The Post-Standard

Chapter 10

OTHER MEMORABLE CASES

Between 1958 and 1972, I conducted hundreds of heart surgeries at St. Joseph's Hospital in Syracuse. These are a few more of my most memorable patients that illustrate the variety and intensity of the cases done during this era.

On April 27, 1960, I was in the doctor's room while waiting to start a case, when I received an urgent call to one of the rooms for a cardiac arrest. The patient was 62-year-old C. D., who had been anesthetized for dental extractions and suddenly went into cardiac arrest. With sterile gloves and skin prep of the chest to provide a sterile field, I performed a left anterior chest incision between the fifth and sixth ribs and a feeble ineffective heart action was noted. Cardiac massage was initiated using both hands and the heart resuscitated immediately. Total time of arrest was one minute. While the incision was closed, the oral surgeon, Dr. Michael Fallon, extracted the upper teeth as planned. The recovery was uneventful, however Mr. D. related in detail of seeing his two brothers, who had died some years before, during surgery. He was overjoyed and did not want to leave them but was awakened in the recovery room.

Interestingly, shortly thereafter, while I was inserting a pacemaker in the cardiopulmonary lab, the elderly female patient had a cardiac arrest. She was shortly resuscitated without difficulty and recovered. During her first post-operative visit she told her family about her "out of body experience." Apparently, she observed me from the ceiling while performing the surgery.

There is no question in my mind that such experiences occur.

J. B. underwent open heart surgery using hypothermia at age 23 for a congenital heart condition, pulmonic valvular stenosis. Her mother was told by doctors that she would not survive to adulthood. She did, and although developed heart failure with her first pregnancy. Her delivery was uneventful. She was next seen by cardiologist Dr. Asher Black, who referred her to Dr. Gensini. A heart catheterization revealed a dynamic pulmonic stenosis and she underwent successful heart surgery in 1962.

In 2008, she emailed me that she had gone on to have two more children, eight grandchildren, and two great grandchildren. "It has been a little over 46 years and still no problems with the surgery. I want you to know how much I appreciate your dedication. Your skilled hands have given me a full life," she wrote.

J. A. was a 29-year-old man who underwent division of a large patent ductus arteriosis with pulmonary hypertension using surface hypothermia in 1965. Normally, the patent ductus between the aorta and pulmonary artery spontaneously seals shortly after birth. When this does not occur, a very high blood pressure develops over the years in the pulmonary arteries, resulting in these vessels becoming thick walled and brittle and extremely difficult to handle. The patient did satisfactorily until his third day post-op, when sudden shock occurred. An emergency thoracotomy (opening of the chest) was done and the bleeding site at the aortic suture line was found and controlled by wrapping the aorta with teflon felt. Felt was used rather than sutures because sutures would only have intensified the bleeding site. His post-op course was thereafter satisfactory and when seen six months later, he had made a remarkable improvement post-operatively.

This case illustrates the disadvantage in not correcting a congenital defect at a much earlier age. By age 29, there are serious changes in the blood vessel walls which make them very friable. A teflon felt wrapping was used to reinforce the suture line as it was deemed much safer than revising the extremely weak aortic wall.

M. K. dated her symptoms of angina to 1968 following a chest injury. Heart catheterization at St. Joseph's on February, 1971, revealed 90 percent obstruction of the right coronary, a complete occlusion of the left anterior descending (LAD) distal to the first septal, and 50 percent obstruction of the diagonal branch. Six months later, at age 55, a bypass vein graft to the right coronary and a left internal mammary implant to the anterolateral wall of the left ventricle were done. Surgery was conducted without the use of the Heart-Lung machine (on pump standby) because there was little or no blood flow through the right coronary artery and there are significant side effects from use of the Heart-Lung machine.

A postoperative study nearly a year later revealed excellent filling of the vein graft to the right coronary and good collateralization of the internal mammary to the distal anterior descending. The left ventricular hemodynamics were normal. She had an excellent course thereafter and was last seen 14 years post-op at age 69, with diabetes.

W. B. was a 35-year-old man who had a saphenous vein bypass from the aorta to the right coronary artery and a left internal mammary implant for severe coronary artery disease. The vein graft occluded at the coronary anastomosis but, left internal mammary artery remained patent and functioning. Five months post-op, the aortic end of the saphenous graft was patent and healthy. The coronary artery connection was occluded. This latter segment of the vein was excised and an additional saphenous vein graft was used to connect the retained graft to a new anastomosis with the right coronary.

Five years post-operatively his condition was excellent and he was playing volleyball four hours a day.

F. C. had an amazing medical history. At age 63, he was first seen in surgical heart consultation by Dr. Anthony Coriale of Utica, New York, with a nine-year history of angina and at least two heart attacks. He had not worked for nine years. Heart catheterization at St. Joe's on December 15, 1971, revealed a significant block in his left coronary artery with good left ventricular function. Symptoms of chest pain increased and surgery was recommended. On March 22, 1972, a bypass with the left internal mammary artery to the left anterior descending coronary was performed. He had an excellent result. Six years later, a pacemaker was implanted for bradycardia (slow heart rate) and in1982, a broken pacer wire was repaired. He had a new pacemaker implanted in 1988.

Later that year, 16 years post bypass, he was

hospitalized for congestive heart failure, SA node syndrome (syndrome with bradycardia) and organic brain dysfunction at age 79. His case was likely the first arterio-coronary bypass in Syracuse and marked the use of arteries rather than veins as conduits, if possible.

R. T. was 26 when he was admitted in the early morning of April 29, 1970, to St. Joseph's emergency room with a history of severe steering wheel injury. X-rays and angiography (dye injected into the blood vessels with x-rays taken) confirmed a ruptured thoracic aorta at the usual site opposite the ligamentum arteriosum (site of former patent ductus). There were also multiple bilateral rib fractures. He was taken immediately to the operating room. A scheduled heart bypass case was canceled and the heart-lung machine was already at readiness.

At surgery there was complete transection of the media and intima of the aorta; the intact adventitia alone prevented a massive lethal exsanguination (blood loss). The aorta has three layers, intima, media and adventitia. The tear was one inch below the subclavian artery. Through a left thoracotomy and partial bypass the transection was repaired by interposing a deacron tube graft to connect the divided aortic ends. His post-op course was uneventful with full recovery.

Chapter 11

STAYING CURRENT

While at a surgical meeting in 1966, Dr. Bob Riemer, a good friend and chest surgeon, and a resident in surgery at the Rhode Island Hospital when I was interning, commented on a new procedure. It was called mediastinoscopy, and consisted of a two-inch horizontal incision in the low neck with dissection along the trachea (windpipe) down to its division into the left and right bronchi. Its purpose is to search for and biopsy lymph nodes for microscopic examination. This is done mainly for lung diseases that often drain into the mediastinal lymph nodes.

The mediastinum is the chest area between the lungs containing the heart, trachea and its division, esophagus, and other smaller but, important structures, including lymph nodes. Such a procedure is valuable for many reasons, but chiefly for the diagnosis of lung cancer. If these nodes are positive, the cancer is inoperable. It is also valuable in diagnosing other non-malignant conditions such as sarcoidosis.

I talked with Bob after the meeting as I had been unfamiliar with the procedure. Bob quipped that I was getting behind times! Needless to say, the next week I visited him in Providence and learned the technique from an expert. Sister Elaine ordered the special equipment necessary.

On returning to Syracuse, I was soon performing mediastinoscopies and subsequently did hundreds with excellent results, extremely low morbidity, and no mortality. This procedure significantly reduced the number of unnecessary chest operations and became a routine pre-operative diagnostic study. It's just one example of the importance of staying current with new procedures and techniques that rapidly evolve in every specialty of medicine.

In 1968, I was accepted as a fellow in the prestigious American College of Cardiology in New Orleans, Louisiana, and could now add FACC to my name.

Despite the credential, progress in technique and technology in open heart surgery was near constant and keeping current was imperative. I traveled a great deal to learn, including visits to Houston, Texas to observe Drs. DeBakey and Cooley, and to the Mayo Clinic, Columbia Medical Center, Georgetown Medical Center, and the Cleveland Clinic. In my view, it was the only way to remain current in this very rapidly developing field. That is what Dr. John Grow used to do.

Unquestionably, there were two most impressive

experiences that I had in that regard.

In the early 70s, while attending a thoracic cardiovascular surgical meeting in Houston, Texas, I joined an informal group of colleagues to visit two nearby adjacent hospitals. There, the two most well known heart surgeons in the entire world, Drs. Michael E. DeBakey and Denton A. Cooley separately worked.

Dr. DeBakey, eight weeks short of 100 years of age at his death in 2008, was a genius. His parents were Lebanese and he was raised and educated in New Orleans, including Tulane University Medical School and surgical residency at Charity Hospital. Following this he spent two years in Europe training under several eminent surgeons. He returned to Tulane, and in 1958 was appointed head of the new Department of Surgery at Baylor University College of Medicine, in Houston, Texas. His early staff included Dr. Cooley. With the advent of cardiopulmonary bypass, DeBakey introduced many innovative cardiovascular techniques, including the first successful aortic aneurysm resection with artificial graft replacement. In addition, he traveled throughout the world performing heart surgery, including on the premier of Russia.

In 1948, Dr. Denton Cooley joined DeBakey in Houston as one of his very first staff members. Dr. Cooley had attended John's Hopkins Medical School and took his surgical residency there. He spent time in England in further surgical training before returning to the U.S. and joining Dr. DeBakey. It was early recognized that he possessed special surgical talents. His techniques were so superior that colleagues who had trained with him would caution those attending surgical meetings not to attempt certain procedures Cooley had reported because they were technically too difficult for most thoracic surgeons.

Needless to say, the team of DeBakey and Cooley did not endure, and in 1969, Dr. Cooley resigned from the full-time faculty at Baylor. Thereafter, each did his surgery at separate hospitals and did not communicate. At the Houston meeting, I attended Dr. Cooley's surgery at St. Luke's Hospital. He was a tremendous showman, extroverted, and enjoyed relating to others. In retrospect, it seems that much of the performance that we witnessed had been planned in conjunction with the meeting. He used three operating rooms with separate teams of well-trained surgeons to assist him. He rotated through the three rooms performing difficult heart operations as his teams opened and closed the chest incisions.

One procedure was a repair of a coarctation of the aorta, which is a congenital marked narrowing of the largest artery in the body. It requires excising this area and connecting the two ends. This required less than one hour total. I had observed the same procedure at Boston Children's

Hospital by a world famous surgeon and it required more than three hours. In addition, the remaining cases required the heart-lung machine. They totaled four in all and were completed within four hours. During the "show," Dr. Cooley allowed us to freely move about in his operating rooms and engaged us in conversation. There was music in the background and he whistled at times!

Following this, I visited Dr. DeBakey at the adjacent Methodist Hospital. The atmosphere was completely the opposite. No visitors were allowed in the operating room and only one room was used. One observed the surgery through a glassed-in observation area. There was no sound except an occasional remark by Dr. DeBakey to the O.R. personnel. Needless to say, his surgery was excellent.

Dr. DeBakey continued in his 90s. In 2006, at age 98, he experienced an extremely serious condition that he himself had researched and treated successfully, a thoracic dissecting ascending aortic aneurysm. It is fatal unless surgery is done and even with surgery, the mortality is high in most circles. He delayed surgery for a day, but then consented and was successfully operated by one of his very capable associates whom he had trained.

After four decades of silence, these two greats mended their rift and in October 2007, Dr. DeBakey was inducted into the Denton A. Cooley Cardiovascular Surgical Society. In

May 2008, Dr. Cooley was inducted into the Michael E. DeBakey International Surgical Society. At that meeting Dr. DeBakey acknowledged Dr. Cooley's considerable contributions to cardiovascular surgery, adding "I don't think I could have done it without Dr. Cooley. In fact I know I couldn't." One week earlier Dr. DeBakey received the Congressional Gold Medal, Congress' highest civilian award. Dr. Cooley did attended the ceremony in Washington, DC.

My experience at the Mayo Clinic was also extremely impressive but in a less dynamic manner. St. Joseph's Hospital had purchased the Mayo Gibbons heart-lung machine. It was the first artificial heart-lung used by Dr. Gibbons in Philadelphia and was further improved at the Mayo Clinic. This clinic is located in the small town of Rochester, Minnesota. It is in the middle of nowhere, however it is an extremely impressive entity in so many ways. I am so convinced that this clinic is so self- sustaining that anything can be produced there.

The person responsible for developing the open heart surgical program at Mayo was Dr. John Kirklin. He was a local product, the son of the chief of radiology at the clinic. John Kirklin was extremely bright and surgically capable. He was a quiet individual whose deeds spoke for themselves. As noted elsewhere, I later personally became more involved with him when he moved to the University of Alabama

Medical Center in Birmingham as Director of Surgery. In addition to his surgical expertise he was a humble man who related in an exceptional manner with his patients. I know because those whom I referred to him--and all were extremely ill--did well surgically and also appreciated his personal touch.

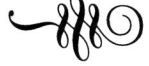

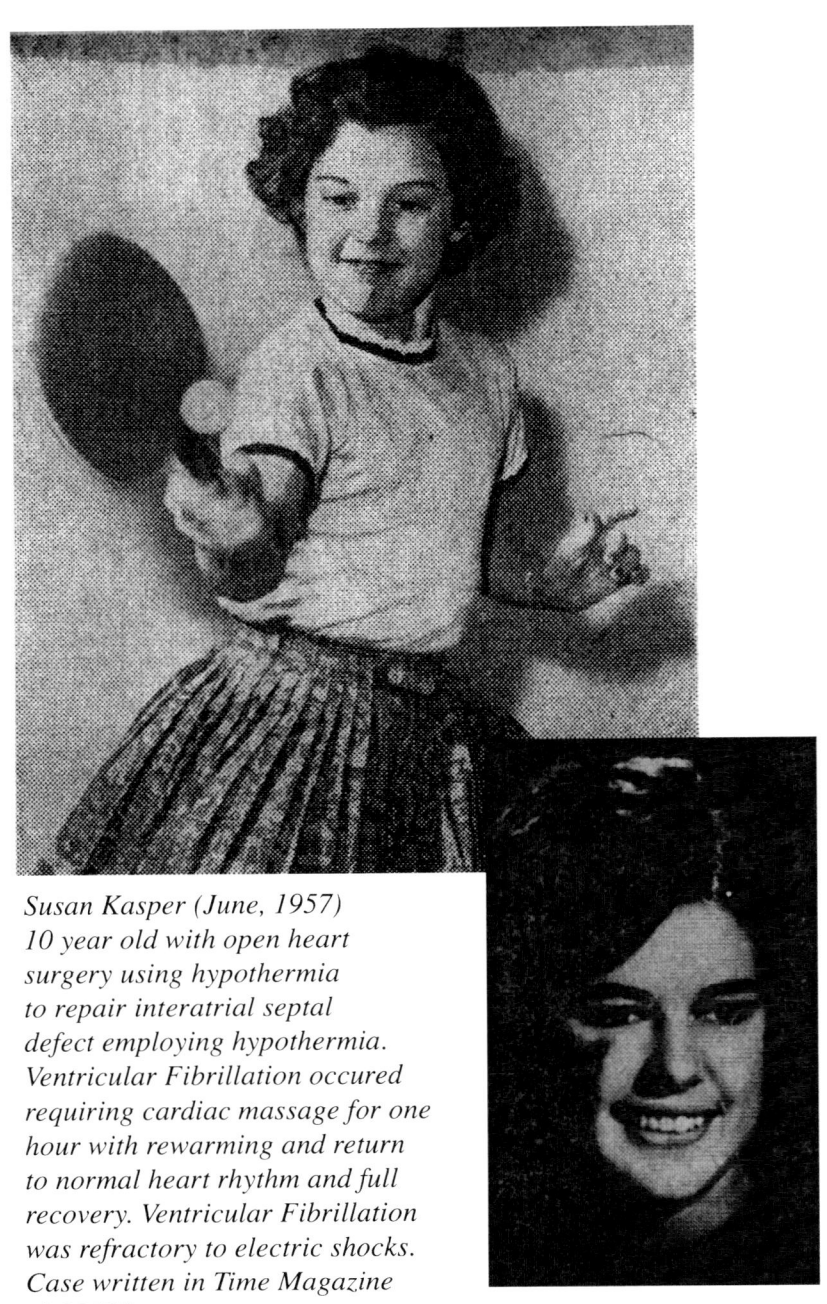

Susan Kasper (June, 1957)
10 year old with open heart
surgery using hypothermia
to repair interatrial septal
defect employing hypothermia.
Ventricular Fibrillation occured
requiring cardiac massage for one
hour with rewarming and return
to normal heart rhythm and full
recovery. Ventricular Fibrillation
was refractory to electric shocks.
Case written in Time Magazine
(9/30/57).

Susan Kasper 13 years later.

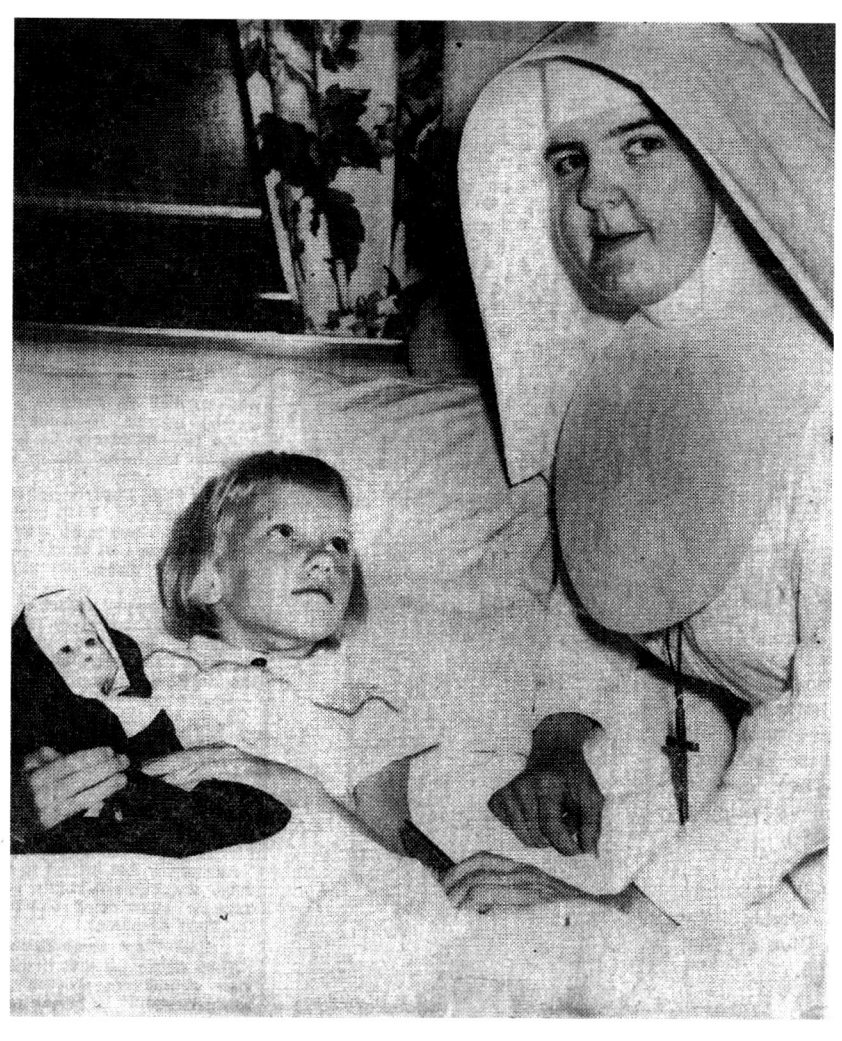

Shown with Sister Julia is 5 yr. old Cheryl Darrat.
At St. Joseph's Hospital Cheryl underwent open heart surgery for a
heart defect. Her heart stopped beating for 10 minutes during her
surgery. Using a new method to get her heart beating again, surgeons
saved her life with full recovery.

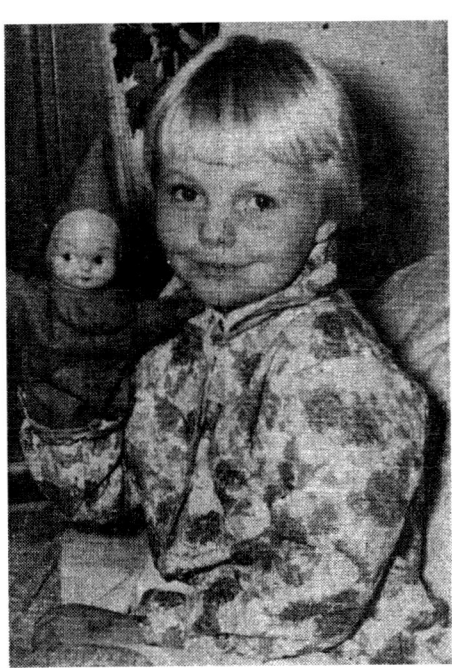

1958
8 year old Sharon Melfi is the first
successful open heart surgery
patient in Syracuse.

In 1986, she graduated from the
Crouse Irving Memorial School
of Nursing. "Yes," she said,
"there is a connection between
making medical history and
choosing a career. Definetely".

Hospital history beats in her
heart - Monday, May 9, 1994
Herald Journal

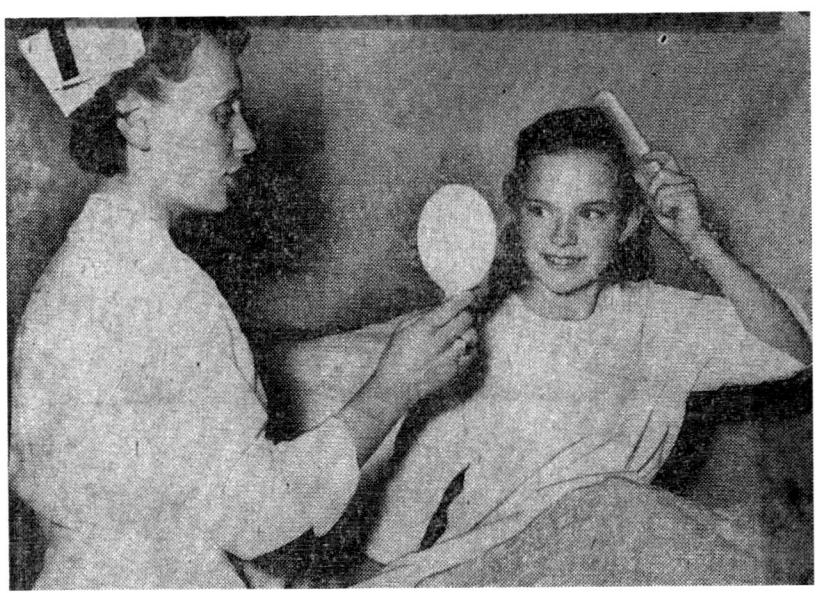

Paula O'Connell (Dec. 1958)
10 year old underwent open heart surgery using hypothermia with
repair of interatrial septal defect with full recovery. Second open
heart surgery in Syracuse.

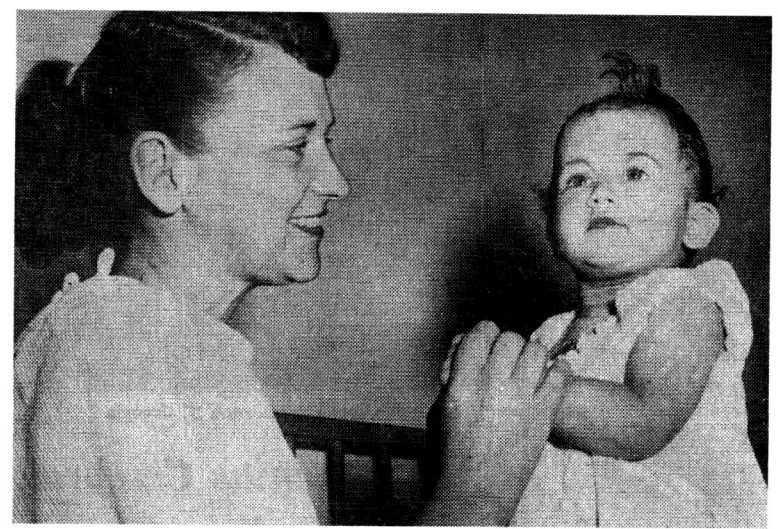

Diane DeBartolo (9/10/59)
10 month old underwent open heart surgery with hypothermia and valvulotomy for pulmonic stenosis.

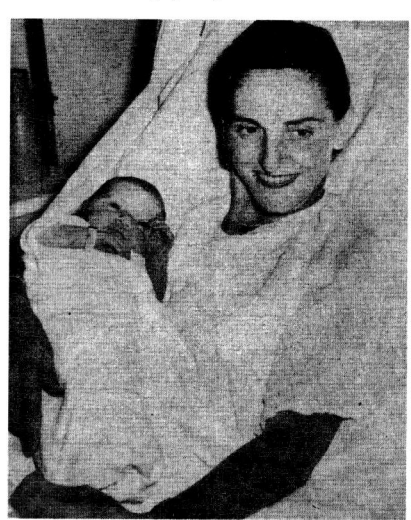

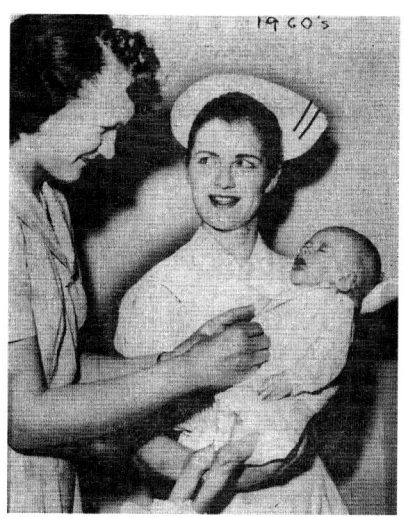

Cynthia Ingles (4/7/60)
Open heart surgery with opening of a narrowed aortic valve in her 8th month of pregnancy.

"Tiny Tim" Fuller (1960)
Blind from cataracts at birth, heart failure at age 3 weeks. At age 4 months division between aorta and pulmonary artery corrected. Heart Failure returned and pulmonic valvulotomy for stenosis with recovery.

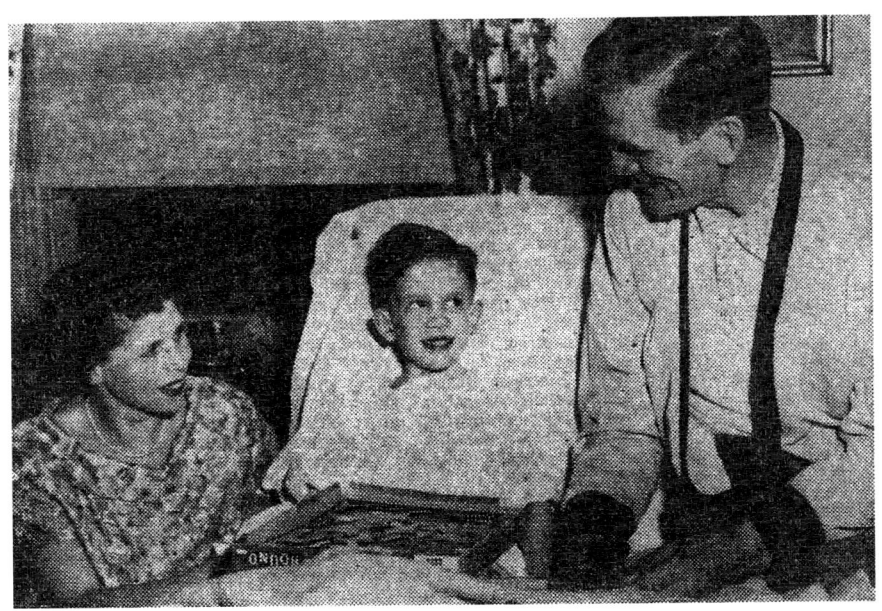

Mike Glavin (4/14/60)
5 year old with correction of congenital pulmonic stenosis using
hypothermia. He became a police officer like his father.

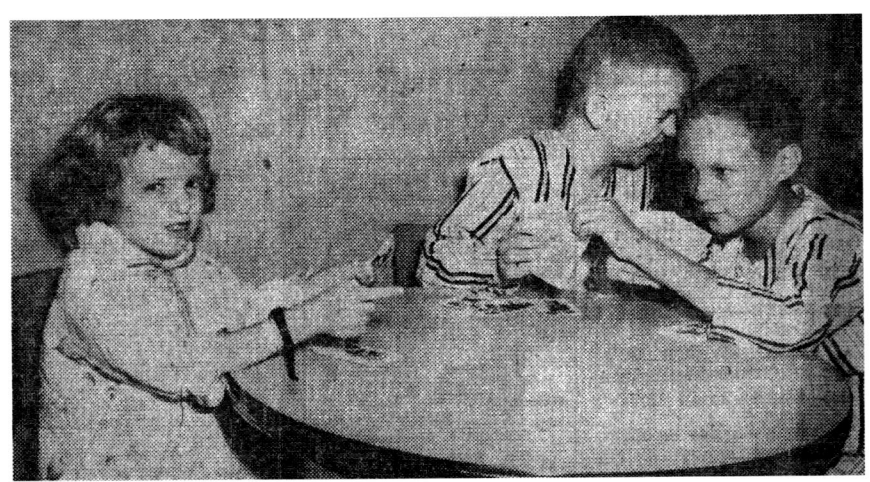

John Thompson, Dale Vanderwater (10/4/61)
Both 9 years old with primum type interatrial septal defects repaired
using the new heart-lung machine. Arlene Schmidt 6 years of age
correction of pulmonic valvular stenosis with hypothermia.

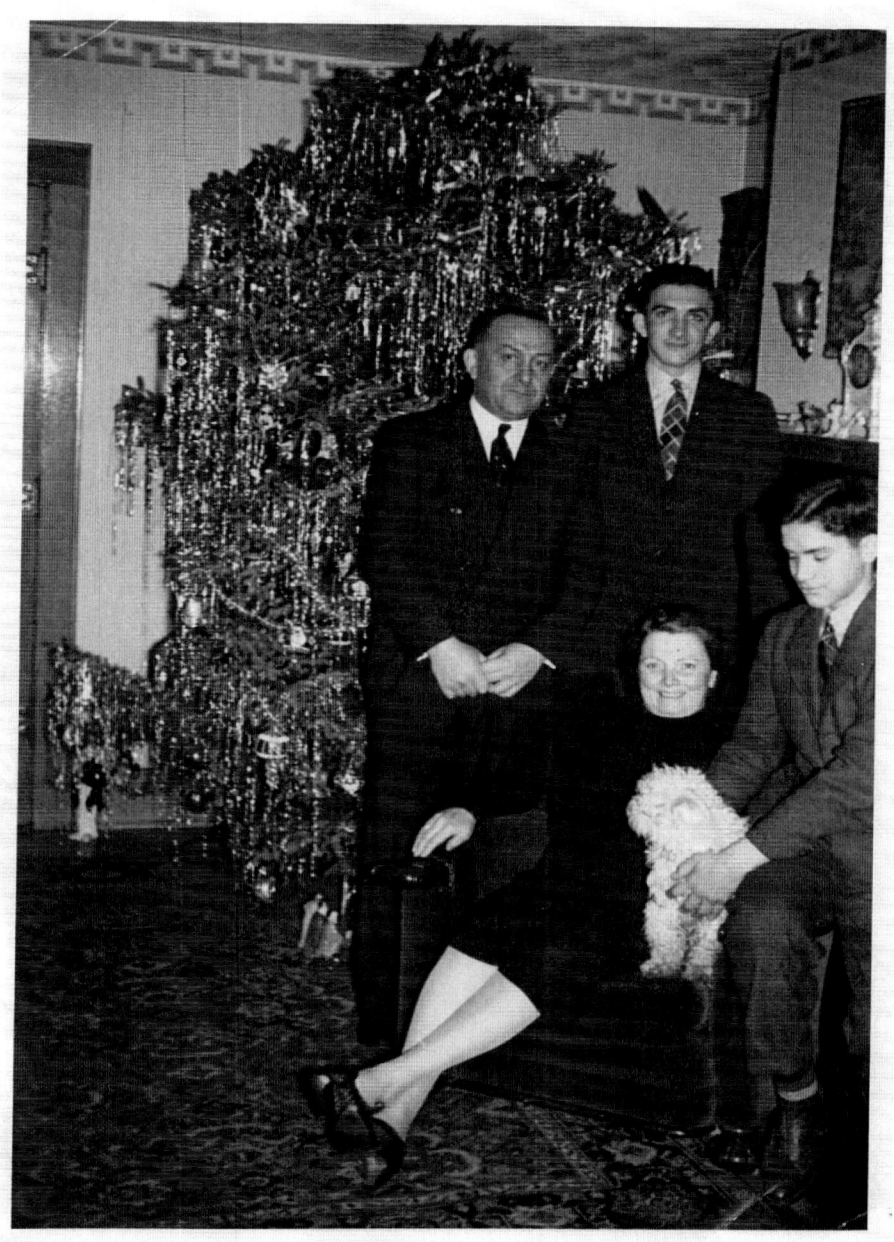

Christmas 1939
Mom, Dad, Jim, Me (16 years old) & Snowball

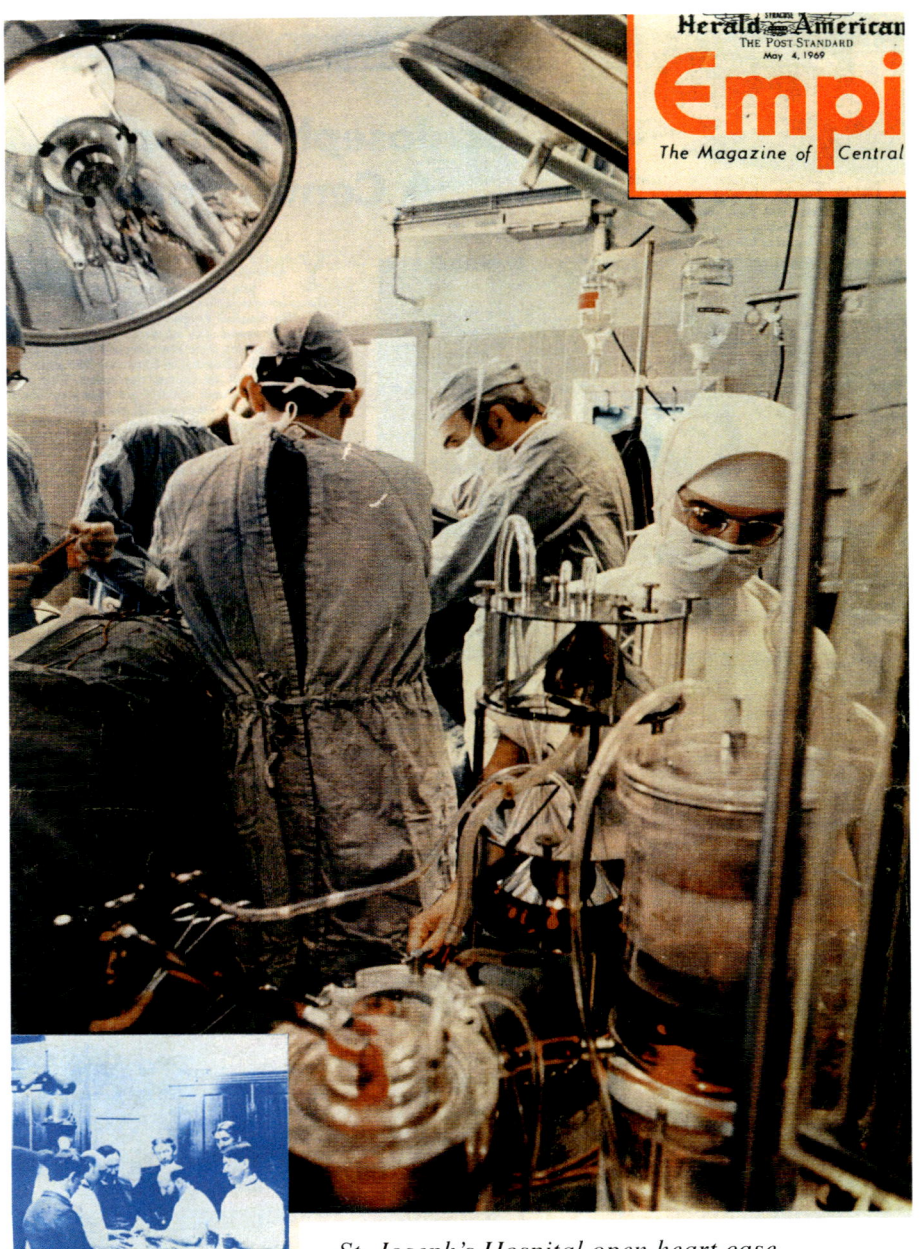

Herald American
THE POST STANDARD
May 4, 1969
Empi
The Magazine of Central

St. Joseph's Hospital open heart case.
Dr. George Heitzman & assistants
Dr. K.S. Rao, Dr. Kato & Sister Laurine
managing the Mayo-Gibbon heart-lung
machine.

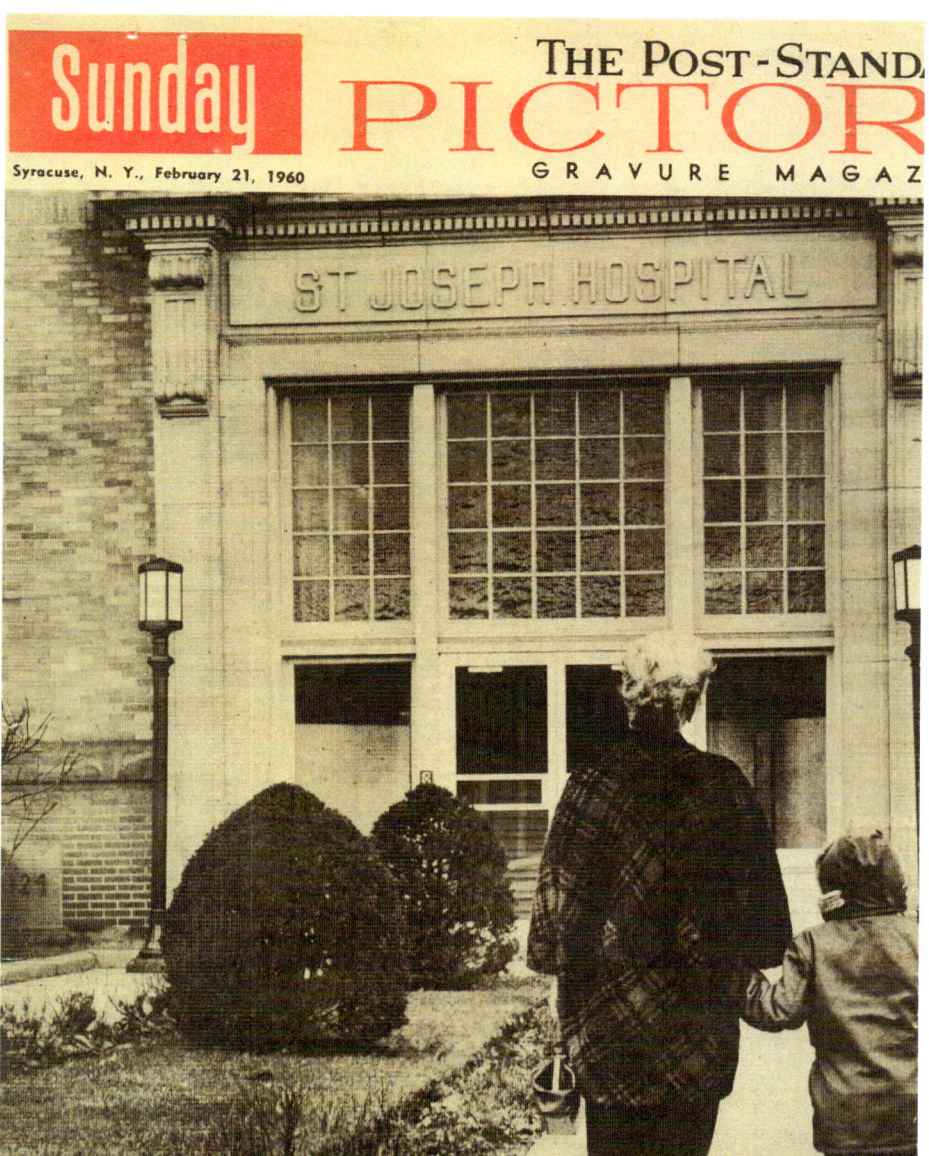

Sunday

THE POST-STAND

PICTOR

GRAVURE MAGAZ

Syracuse, N. Y., February 21, 1960

*Large article concerning open heart surgery at St. Joseph's Hospital.
Young Mike McMahon with his mother entering the hospital on the day
of his surgery.*

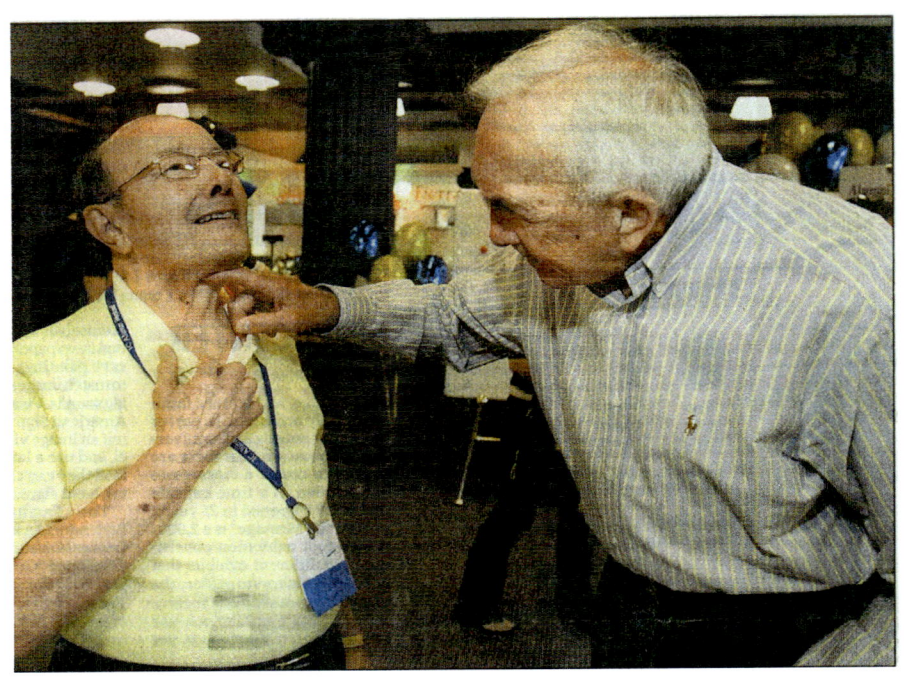

St. Joseph's Hospital open heart case.
Joe Palmieri (left) shows his heart surgery scar to the man who gave it to
him 39 years ago, Dr. George Heitzman at Ithaca College where Palmieri
was attending his 55th class reunion.

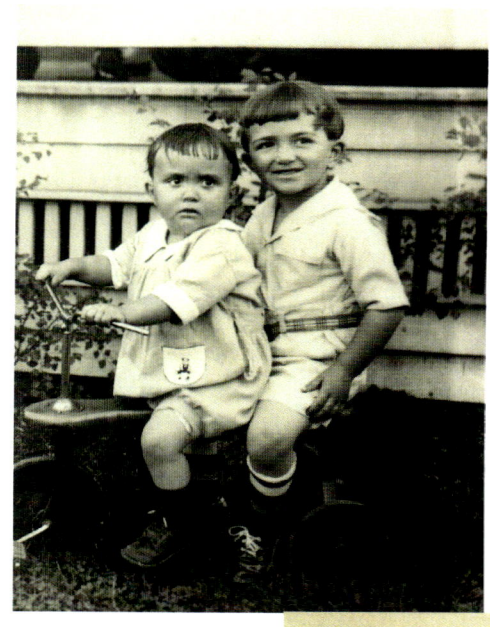

Brother Jim and I as young boys.

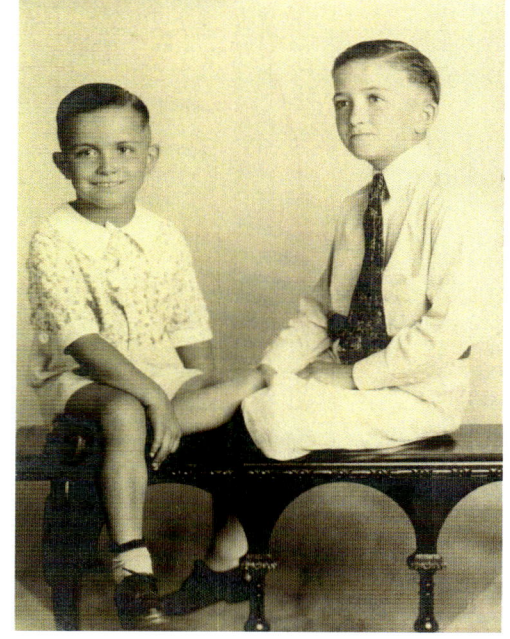

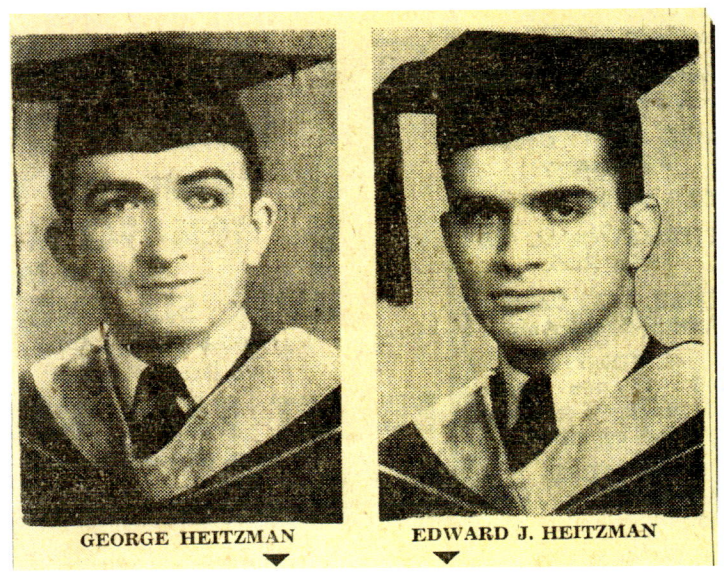

GEORGE HEITZMAN   EDWARD J. HEITZMAN

Brother Jim and I receive M.D. degrees in 1947.

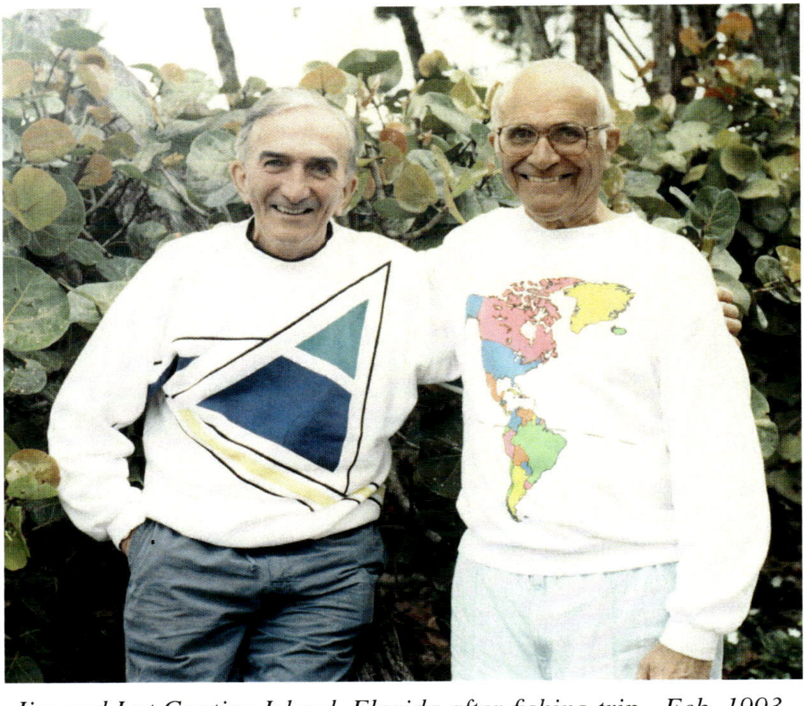

Jim and I at Captiva Island, Florida after fishing trip - Feb. 1993

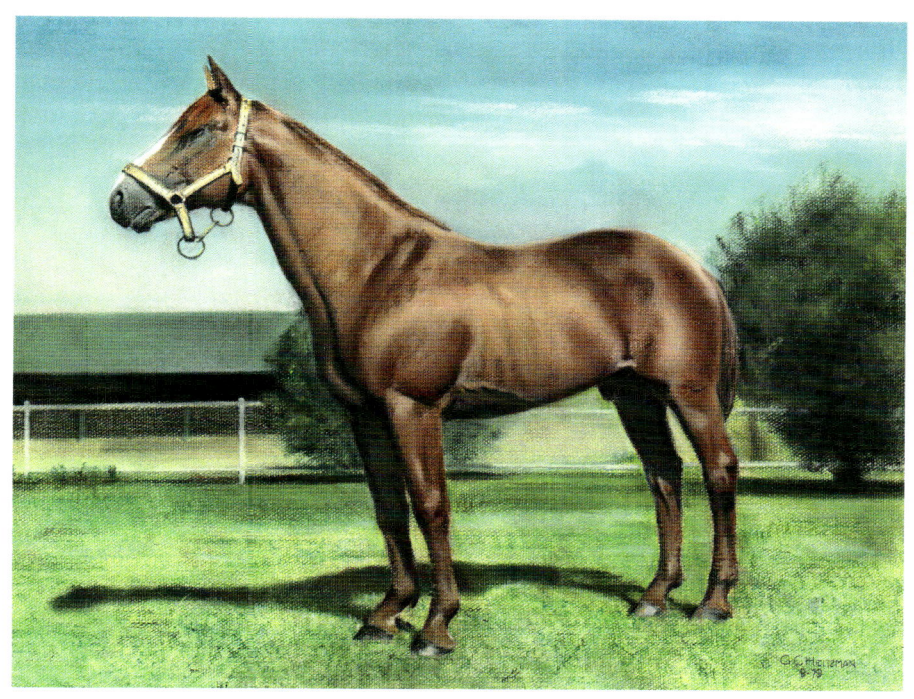

Sophora
Champion Trotter
Pastel by George Heitzman

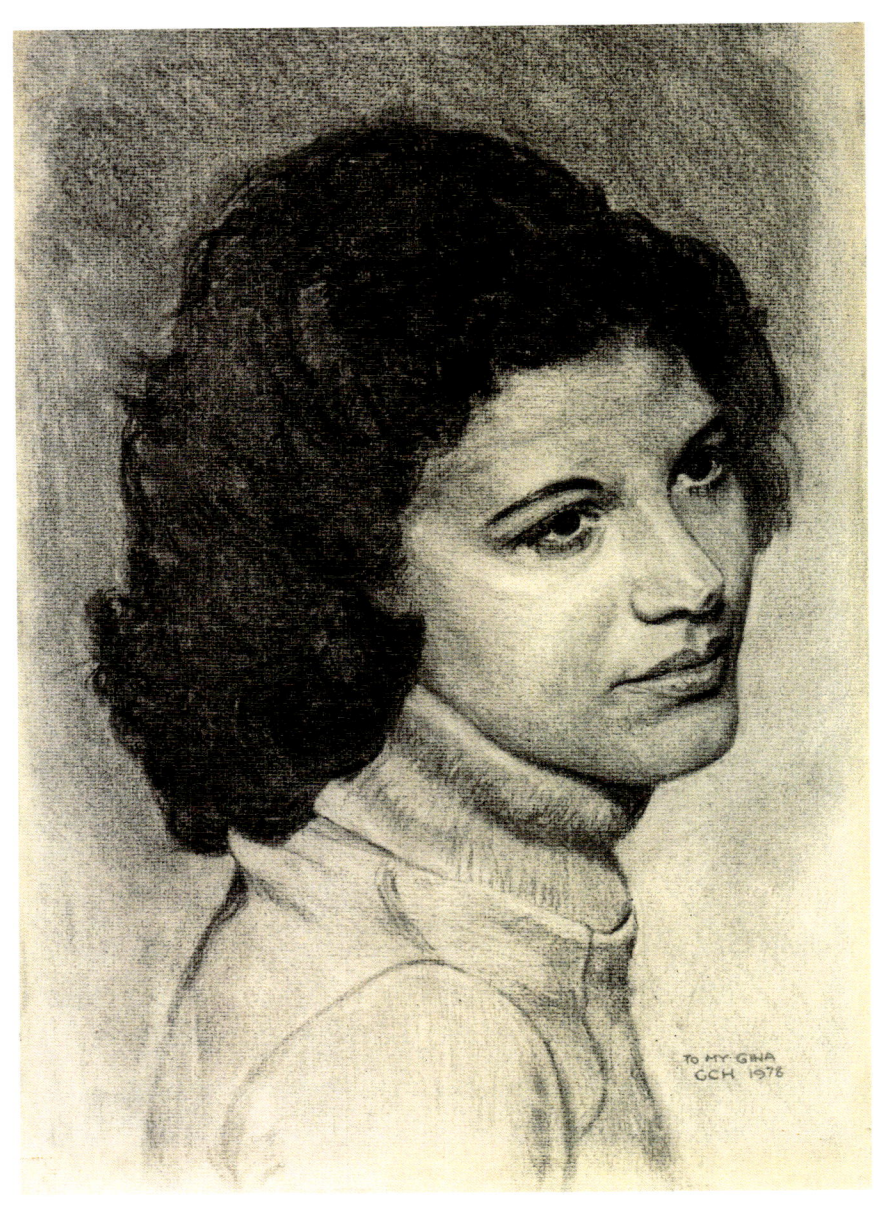

Gina
Charcoal by George Heitzman

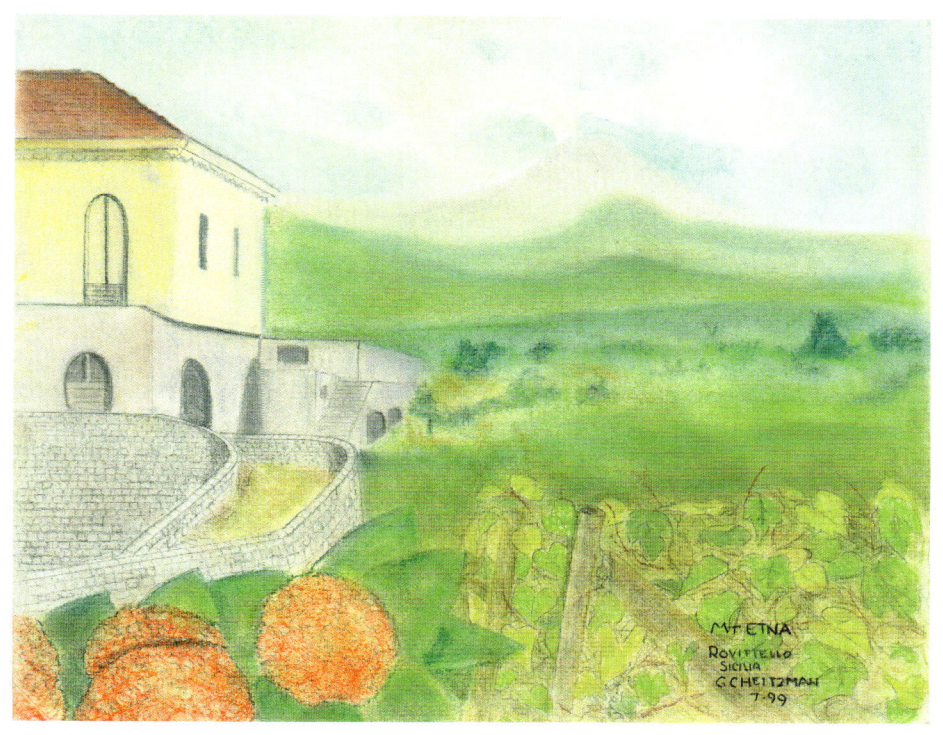

Mt. Etna
Rovittello, Sicily
Pastel by George Heitzman

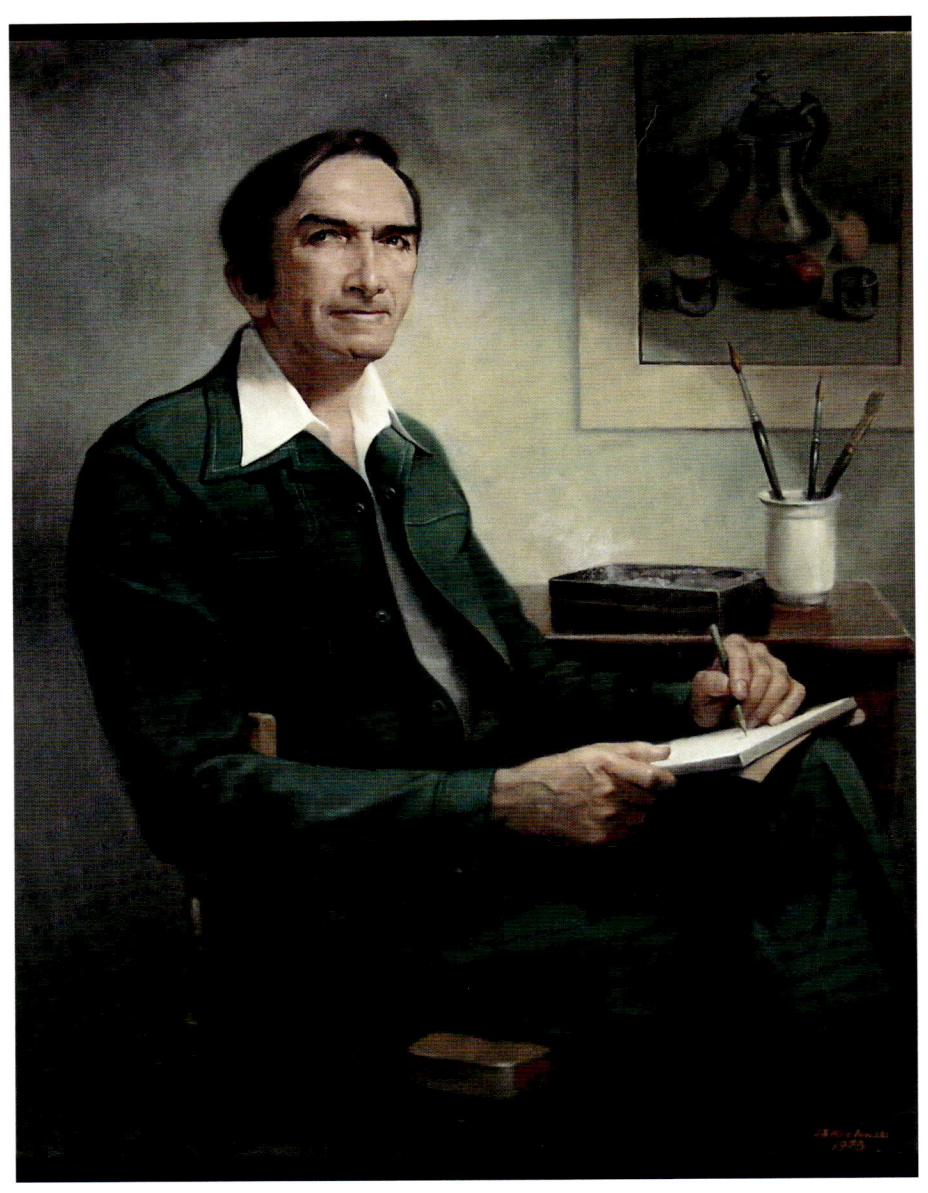

Portrait of George Heitzman
Oil
Artist: Joe Kozlowski - 1978

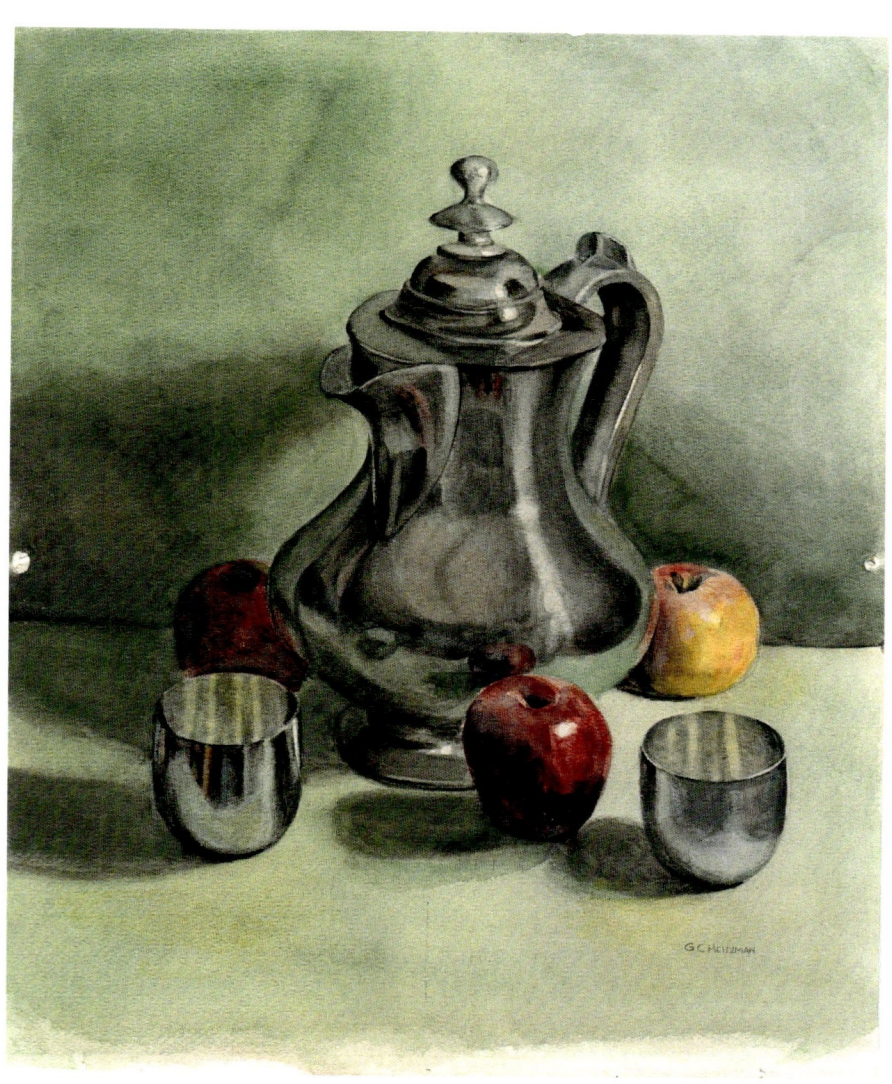

Watercolor by George Heitzman

Chapter 12

A DIFFICULT TURNING POINT

In the 1970s, I personally experienced many challenges and it is difficult to weigh the importance of them individually.

Surgical fees allowed by insurance for heart surgeons were relatively low as compared with other surgery, when years of training required are considered. This never changed during my career. All open heart surgery at St. Joseph's while I was active included both Dr. Delmonico and myself. This was indeed a great advantage to the patient, who had the benefit of two experienced thoracic surgeons working together throughout the entire surgical procedure. We always equally divided the total surgical fees.

Personally, I could not have made a living on heart surgery alone, as at most I performed one open heart case a week. The remaining thoracic surgery provided by far the majority of my income. Open heart surgery was done because I loved it and derived great personal satisfaction from it.

Our open heart program had progressed well, though we had not increased the volume beyond one weekly for 12 years when the first coronary artery bypass was successfully performed in 1970 at St. Joseph's Hospital. This type of surgery opened up a huge demand because of the volume of patients in need of the procedure.

Direct surgery on the coronary arteries is extremely intricate as the obstructed arteries measured 2 to 4mm in diameter.(24 mm equals 1 inch) and the suturing to bypass arteries with grafts 4 mm in diameter required very fine 5-0 sutures with the use of magnifying lens. These were very difficult surgical procedures and required more than one case every two weeks to attain and maintain suitable surgical proficiency. This was extremely important to the patient as well as the surgeon. By comparison, large volume centers, such as the Mayo Clinic, were conducting approximately nine coronary bypass procedures a day at that time.

Sister Wilhelmina, always a longtime supporter of the open heart program, had become seriously ill, necessitating her resignation as administrator. I went to the new hospital administrator in 1972 and explained the necessity of increasing the number of open heart surgeries per week.

He immediately answered that it was impossible because there would not be sufficient ICU beds for one year!

Admittedly, I was bewildered by this response but set off to find areas suitable for more ICU beds. Though I found a number of areas I felt were feasible, but all were rejected.

Next I contacted Dr. Delmonico, and we met privately in a restaurant on Erie Boulevard. I explained my position about the urgent need for more coronary heart surgery at St. Joe's and suggested that we meet together with administration and be more demanding in our requests, suggesting that we would threaten to stop all open heart operations if they did not agree. He said very little but that he could not stop performing heart surgery. There was no explanation for his decision.

Admittedly, I was very surprised and extremely disappointed. I left him at the restaurant and shortly afterward informed all concerned, including my referring doctors, that I had discontinued all open heart surgery. I just didn't see how I could maintain the skill level necessary attempting to perform sophisticated procedures at such a low volume.

My patients always came first and I was not willing to put them in jeopardy for the sake of my ego. My dreams for the open heart surgery program at St. Joseph's were crumbling.

Withdrawing from the program I had planned and worked so hard to build was one of the most difficult decisions of my life. The program largely existed due to the presence of Sister Wilhelmina and her desire to fill a community need not available elsewhere between Rochester and Albany. After her death in early 1977, many significant changes ensued at St. Joseph's. Structural changes took place, including demolition of the beautiful chapel frequented by many patients, relatives, and hospital personnel. Some felt that when the chapel was destroyed, it became a symbol of a much different philosophy.

One year after I withdrew from the program I created, the open heart surgical program at St. Joe's ceased, but not before a young heart surgeon joined Dr. Delmonico.

Dr. M. Zafrullah Kahn, a capable young heart surgeon from Atlanta, Georgia, joined Dr. Delmonico in 1973. A new Sarnes heart-lung machine was purchased to replace the Mayo-Gibbon. Apparently it was much more practical. It could be cleaned rapidly and used several times a day. Dr. Delmonico assisted Dr. Kahn with the surgery. This association was short lived, however. I heard from several sources there was disagreement between them.

In 1974 a cardiologist approached and asked if I had an interest in returning to heart surgery and working with the new young surgeon. I told him I would think it over.

In December 1974, an internist-friend contacted me and asked if I would consult on a 57- year-old-male with an acute dissecting aneurysm of the ascending aorta who was just admitted as an emergency patient. I did so, and then asked Dr. Kahn if he was interested in consulting on this case and performing the emergency bypass surgery. He was, and I assisted him with the procedure.

The patient's condition was extremely serious with a poor known prognosis at that time. The patient expired in the operating room. Shortly thereafter, Dr. Kahn moved out of town.

In the meantime, Upstate Medical Center had developed an open heart program. Dr. Fritz Parker shortly emerged as the chief of cardio-thoracic surgery and then director of the department of surgery. Fritz was a very capable surgeon in all respects and ran an excellent thoracic surgery residency program.

The original open heart surgical program in Syracuse started in 1958 and ceased in 1974, although I left in 1972. In 1978, Dr. Donald Effler arrived with his team to re-start the open heart program at St. Joseph's to much fanfare. Due to the resources provided, the program was successful. Dr. Effler was referred to as the "god" by many involved, a title he appeared to enjoy.

I would not be honest if I did not admit that this was difficult for me. I never understood the politics that prevented such support for my program in earlier years and my resentment was misplaced toward the new regime.

Tragically, the end of Dr. Effler's life was very sad. He spent many months in a nursing home forgotten by those same people that had idolized him.

I decided to set aside my anger and visit him. His nurses mentioned that he had very few to no visitors. I do not believe that he was mentally intact during this encounter, but I felt a definite exhilaration at letting go of my resentment. I was at peace.

The lack of support to expand the open heart program at a critical juncture—only to see it emerge just a few years later—had been a lifelong thorn. If I were paranoid, I might think efforts were in motion to thwart the program from the time it was initiated by Sister Wilhelmina. There must have been dissidents to her plan, although I was never directly aware of them during my 14 years of heart surgery.

This frustration was compounded through the years by a seeming disregard for history. In 2006, the Onondaga County Medical Society published *The History of Local Medical Care, 1806-2006: Celebrating Physicians Past and Present*. It includes no mention of the first open heart surgery program or laboratory in Syracuse.

The following year, St. Joseph's Hospital and Health Center devoted an issue of its newsmagazine *Caring Connection* to cardiac surgery at the institution. Aside from a small mention of Sharon Melfi as the first open heart patient in 1958, there were no mentions of the origins of the program. Were readers to think that the open heart program actually began in 1982 and ignore Melfi in 1958?

I feel privileged to have had a role in a unique piece of Syracuse medical history and there were many selfless personalities who were integral in their participation. My goal in writing this memoir has never been to detract from others achievements but to document history and put closure to an important part of my life.

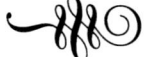

Chapter Thirteen

THOUGHTS OF MOVING WEST

In 1972, after deciding to stop performing open heart surgery at St. Joseph's Hospital, I gave very serious consideration to moving west and to continue with it at a hospital with greater surgical volume. I considered Colorado, New Mexico, and Utah, and visited hospitals in each state.

Denver was the only place I had some familiarity with. I stopped at NJH and there was no one left there that I knew. It had been 15 years since my training. All of the familiar medical personnel had left and there were many changes. Surgery was no longer done; the institution was now primarily a medical chest hospital for allergic problems such as asthma, although it was still very well known and highly regarded nationally and internationally.

My friend from France and Iowa City, Dr. Jim Bauer, had left the military years before and taken a radiology residence including radiotherapy. Jim had many hats. He was always an exceptional fellow but he did surprise me when he went into the Episcopalian Seminary and became a priest. His wife Carol was indeed an exception and supported him all the way. They moved to Denver where he functioned both as a minister and part-time radiologist. They invited me to stay with them and their family while in Denver. I looked around at several other hospitals and there were some possibilities. I did see Dr. Grow during my visit.

I realized I had made a good decision not to remain in Denver, although I did receive a medical license in Colorado.

Next I traveled to Santa Fe, New Mexico. The beauty of the Rockies in this area was incredible. Here too, I applied and was granted a state license. Next, I went south to Albuquerque where Dr. Al Chester was practicing surgery and doing very well. He had been a surgical resident at St. Joe's and we had worked together considerably, including cardiac surgery. Al was very obliging and invited me to stay at his home and showed me around the hospitals.

A group of three surgeons were doing open heart surgery successfully. One was from Denver and had worked with Dr. Grow for a short time. It was evident they were a hard-working group but not as well organized as our Syracuse program. Again, I realize this move would not have been successful.

The third visit was to Reno, Nevada, and I was granted licensure after an interview. I then proceeded to Las Vegas. There the other side of the "City of Sin" was revealed to me, the living areas of the employees of the city, including hospitals.

I met the two heart surgeons who were partners. The older was Dr. Harold Feikus, who was very interesting and friendly. He was a Westerner and had his big break when he was summoned in consultation. The patient was the chief lieutenant of the world famous billionaire, Howard Hughes. This man had an abdominal aneurysm about to rupture. Harold made this diagnosis and advised immediate surgery. The patient indicated that he wished to fly to Houston and have the surgery performed by the famous Dr. Michael DeBakey. Harold countered that the aneurysm could rupture in the plane en route. Needless to say, this man remained in Las Vegas for his surgery, which was performed by Dr. Feikus with excellent results. Shortly thereafter Harold was introduced to the famous Howard Hughes and became his physician. This meant that he was on call 24-hours-a-day , seven-days-a-week. Howard was allowed full use of a Hughes private plane. The newspaper heard of this relationship and immediately he was fired.

Of all three visits, Las Vegas was the most promising from the standpoint of being welcomed to come and perform all forms of chest surgery.

But after returning to Syracuse, I realized more and more that I would be leaving a well- established practice and starting all over at age 49. In retrospect this was a very wise decision.

Chapter Fourteen

MY GINA

The 1970s were difficult in many ways and I was not happy.

My dream, the open heart program, ran into an impasse and I felt forced to relinquish it. Although I'd considered relocating, I decided it was too late in my life to start over. Overall, I was discouraged.

One day in 1978, I was leisurely walking about in the operating room waiting to start a case. I happened to look into a room where an abdominal operation was in progress and saw the most beautiful neck I had ever seen on the scrub nurse. She looked up briefly and noted my gaze.

Shortly thereafter we met, but she remained distant and guarded. I found out that she was single, along with being beautiful, and I was aware she had other admirers.

I sent her flowers and that embarrassed her. She told Sister Elaine, the operating room supervisor, thinking this would control any further incidents. Instead, Sister assigned Gina to scrub in and assist on chest surgery every afternoon I operated!

She hadn't known Sister Elaine was a good friend of mine. Although Elaine and I never discussed it, I am forever indebted to this very proper nun who was so bright, deep, and understanding. Many years later, Gina admitted that she had expected Sister Elaine to assign her to Dr. Josh Malgieri's hemorrhoidectomy cases instead!

Gina and I began seeing each other and fell in love. We married on July 25, 1980. I was very blessed to be allowed to marry in the Catholic Church at Our Lady of Pompei Church by Rev. Monsignor Paul Brigandi, who has been a life-long friend, and with a very intimate, elegant wedding reception at the Persian Terrace at the Hotel Syracuse. Debbie Murphy was our matron of honor and Jim Heitzman was my best man.

I appreciated the support given to both Gina and me by Debbie and her husband, attorney Michael, along with her parents and grandparents during the early years of our courtship and marriage when we needed it the most.

We have had a marvelous marriage. Gina went on to graduate from Crouse Irving School of Nursing, as had my mother, and then obtained her baccalaureate and master's degrees in nursing from Syracuse University, with honors. She was an adjunct professor at the Syracuse University College of Nursing until our son, Jacob, arrived in 1988.

Through the years, Gina has been very active in the community, especially with the Onondaga County Medical Society Alliance. She served on the board for 10 years and has held many titles, including president. In 1999, Gina received the Onondaga County Medical Society Alliance Service to the Community Award. In 2002, she was a recipient of the Onondaga County Medical Society Service to the Alliance Award.

She started an after school science club program at Immaculate Conception School where Jake attended elementary school. This was very successful and Gina coordinated all of the science activities and experiments.

Gina has chaired many successful fundraisers that have benefitted numerous nonprofit needy agencies in the community. One that stands out in my mind is fulfilling a Christmas wish list for residents of Mesa Commons and De Palmer House for families, where at least one family member is afflicted with the HIV virus. I recall loading our two SUVs with gifts and delivering them. It was a fulfilling experience for us both.

One of her pet projects was the SAVE Day (Save Our Schools). The poster contest conducted as part of SAVE in local elementary schools was targeted at third graders and was designed as part of an anti-violence initiative. The artwork of the winning posters was published as a calendar, which was made available to schools, families and the community.

We have enjoyed traveling to Europe on several occasions, especially Italy. The country there and its weather, along with the food, have been delightful. Gina is fluent in Italian and this provides me with much security. Gina's family in Sicily has been very warm, welcoming, and hospitable. I have especially enjoyed the fresh fish off the pier and the homemade wine.

I recall on one such visit to Sicily with Santa and Jake where we stayed in Giardini Nexus nestled below the beautiful town of Taormina offering a view of rare beauty of Mt. Etna and the seacoast. The Greek and Roman Theater is the most visited monument, at an unrecorded time the Greeks hewed the theater out of rock on the slope of Mt. Tauro, but the Romans remodeled and modified it greatly for their amusement. The Giardino Pubblico is a lovely flower-filled garden overlooking the sea. Taormina also offers world class hotels, restaurants and shopping.

One evening, while feasting on fresh seafood at the home of Gina's cousin Lucia, we observed Mt. Etna erupting with fire and lava pouring out of the mountain. The lava ash covered the island and delayed our flight the next morning. When we finally took off, the mountain was still erupting as we passed overhead. It is well known that the rich soil of Sicily due to the ash is what produces the special produce including lemons. I enjoyed watching Gina's uncles Francesco and Peppino make their own wine from their vineyards. Gina's father Francesco and his family were in the business of wine making from their vineyards.

She is very close and loyal to her only living parent, Santa, who lives in Syracuse.

Winters are spent in part on Sanibel Island, Florida. We have found this spot to be truly a jewel. The beautiful sea shell beaches are striking. The lack of high rises and low key atmosphere lends itself to a true island experience.

Close friends Tony and Trish Brunsing and Linda and Dave Essig are owners on the island and we spend a great deal of time with them. Tony and Trish have two sons Jacob's age, Brian and Paul, and the three have enjoyed Sanibel together since they were preschoolers. Even today, our fondest times are sitting on the beach sharing memories with Tony and Trish.

Linda was a former patient of mine that I operated on in 1984 and we developed a friendship as couples. We have wonderful memories of past trips with them, including cruises to Europe and the Caribbean. Last winter, we had a pleasurable time with them in Sanibel and returned to Captiva by boat, where I was able to reminisce about the wonderful times I had with my brother.

Linda and Dave presented me with a very special gift that I will always treasure. It is the enlarged article and photo published in the *Post Standard* on June 16, 2008. This was beautifully framed and it hangs in my office today.

Gina and I have lived in the same house since we were married in 1980. It was purchased on Valentine's Day and we have been truly happy here. We have spacious land and are only eight minutes away from St. Joseph's Hospital, where emergency calls were not unusual.

One reason for our happiness here, was our next-door neighbors, the Patils. One day shortly after we moved in, Viji appeared at the door with a large bouquet of peonies to welcome us. One of her many talents is gardening and we have often admired her gardens.

Drs. Patil were born in India where they attended medical school separately. Each of them moved to England for specialty training, Umesh in surgery and Viji in anesthesiology. There, they met, fell in love, and married. They came to the United States and eventually settled in Syracuse, where they both became full-time faculty members at Upstate Medical Center. Both have outstanding careers in their respective specialties.

Umesh has published extensively in pediatric urology, including a method of repairing urethral strictures in males. Viji has similarly contributed to the literature with an ingenious use of magnets in performing bronchoscopies. By magnetizing the tip of the bronchoscope and placing a magnet on the skin surface overlying the larynx, the instrument can readily be passed into the trachea and its divisions.

Padma, their oldest child, graduated from Cornell University, finishing with an MBA. She is very successful in the Syracuse business community. Neena, their youngest child, received her undergraduate degree at Georgetown University and her law degree from the University of Michigan. She is married to Prashanth Jayachandran, a lawyer, and they live in Princeton, New Jersey, with their charming and entertaining young son, Tarak. Their second child, Devan, was born October 21, 2010.

The Patils moved out of the neighborhood to Skaneateles Lake several years ago when Viji retired and we have missed them.

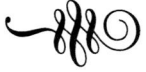

Chapter Fifteen

THE CHILDREN

My commitment to building my career, particularly the open heart program, was not without sacrifice. I had four children during this period that I was able to spend relatively little time with while they were young, largely because of my commitment to my work.

In the 22 years since my retirement, we have attempted to make up for lost time, something Gina has strongly encouraged. I am very proud of all my children and grandchildren:

George, Jr., is a Holy Cross College graduate and a strong Christian. He spends much of his time helping his fellow man here in Syracuse. His daughter Eden, a Princeton graduate, is married to Artur, they have three children.

Donna was a chiropractor in Connecticut and has a fine reputation in her field. She is very personable, entertaining, and sweet. She has recently moved back into the area.

Peter is an extremely popular and fine guitarist. He is married to Karen Savoca, who has a beautiful voice. Together they entertain locally, nationally, and internationally

(Canada).

They write all of their own original music. They are very highly respected in their professions.

They live locally outside of Syracuse in a charming old church house that they renovated and when home love to cook from scratch together.

Jennifer is very gifted artistically and a hard-working homemaker. She is also a great cook and loves to bake. She has a daughter, Jacqueline, who is delightful and now attending college. Jenny is married to a very talented and spiritual man, Paul Brown, and together they are restoring a home in Glens Falls, which is both historical and architecturally beautiful.

Gina and I had our son, Jake, in 1988 and I retired later that year. My retirement provided me the time and joy in raising Jacob with Gina. This included participation in activities including sports, basketball, baseball and golf. We also share a great love and talent for art. Jake graduated from St. Joseph's University in Philadelphia as a Biology major in May, 2010.

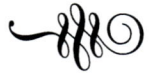

Chapter Sixteen

THORACIC SURGERY

Although my open heart surgical career ended in 1972, I was most fortunate to fulfill this dream. All of my practice has been confined to thoracic surgery and I continued a thriving thoracic surgery practice at St. Joseph's Hospital until my retirement in 1988.

In addition to enjoying the unique and satisfying relationships with my patients, one of the most satisfying aspects of my work was working with residents: furthering their skills, learning from them, and sometimes developing close connections in the process.

Admittedly, I have had favorite residents at St. Joseph's and very, very few poor ones. It does become "tricky" to choose the best.

As a group, those doctors from India stand out, dating back to Murphy David in the 1950s, when we first started the open heart program. He epitomized the qualities these young men brought to St. Joseph's, being polite, courteous, industrious, and very bright.

Dr. Kodem "Samba" Rao was, and always will be, very close to me. After finishing the surgical residency he desired to be a thoracic surgeon. I helped him with a residency in Chicago with Syracuse alum, Dr. Shelley Burman. Upon completing this training, he returned as my partner in private practice. This was in the mid-seventies when I was no longer performing open heart surgery. After approximately a year, he said he would like to train further with Dr. Dudley Johnson of Milwaukee, a superb heart surgeon who popularized the concept of performing multiple vein bypass grafts. (His reasoning was that if one or more grafts obstructed there were still others open. Most heart surgeons adopted his approach.)

I later met Samba at a thoracic meeting in Toronto, Canada, and he flew back to Syracuse with me.

He said that while he was very satisfied with his Milwaukee experience, he wanted to return to be partners again with me even though there would be no open heart surgery.

I was so flattered, but painfully, told him that not realizing his wishes, I had already arranged for Dr. Amilcar Barreto to join me in practice on completion of his thoracic residency at Upstate Medical Center. I continue to feel badly over this. Samba is a very special and capable physician and I feel we would have had a long standing partnership.

Our son Jacob was commissioned into the US Air Force as a Second Lieutenant on graduating from St. Joseph's

University May 15, 2010. He was assigned to the Science Laboratory at Wright Patterson Air Force Base, Dayton, Ohio and recently received orders to report for active duty.

I learned that Dr. K.S. Rao had been practicing heart surgery in the Dayton area and with some difficulty Gina reached him. It was so delightful to talk with him and renew our friendship after 30 years. Gina, Jake and I traveled to Dayton in September 2010 to help him find an apartment and purchase necessities. It was a very successful trip in all respects including an invitation to Liz and Samba's home and having a very delicious meal with them. It was a wonderful evening and we are hopeful of many more. Samba has been very successful as a board certified thoracic and cardiovascular surgeon and recently retired. They have one son, Adam. Seeing him again has meant a great deal to me. He expressed an interest in volunteering his services to India or Africa one month each year. This is so typical of this fine individual.

I have known Dr. Amilcar Barreto since 1969 when he came as an intern and then went through the general surgical residency. He was very bright, knowledgeable and capable. I have known his mother and sister as well and helped him through the years. We were partners for four years after his thoracic residency training and we continue to remain in touch.

Dr. Shreekant Tripathi is still close to my heart. He is such a beautiful person, always pleasant, courteous and good natured. He had a great sense of humor. He was very skilled and competent and helped me operate on Bishop Harrison of Syracuse even though he was not on the chest service, but was chief surgical resident.

One of my classmates and my personal physician for many years, Dr. Carl Austin, shared the same office with Dr. EJ and me. He and my brother were very close friends. Carl was my personal physicians for many years. In April 1981, Carl referred the Roman Catholic Bishop of Syracuse, Frank Harrison, because of a lung mass detected on a routine chest x-ray. He was a non-smoker, always healthy and in his eighties. A work up was done including bronchoscopy and a definite diagnosis could not be made although the findings were consistent with tumor.

Dr. Austin cleared him for lung surgery. On April 17, 1981, a left thoracotomy was performed and an 8 cm. in diameter mass was present in the upper lobe. An upper lobectomy was performed and the postoperative course was uneventful. The pathology report was carcinoid tumor, or adenoma.

These are usually considered benign, but in this case the tumor had invaded an adjacent lymph node. Other lymph nodes were free of disease.

Bishop Harrison lived in good health until age 90. He was a very low key, humble man and highly revered.

Interestingly, the surgery was performed on Good Friday, the day of Christ's crucifixion. It was the first time an elective (non-emergent) operation was done at St. Joseph's Hospital on that day. After the surgery, the Syracuse newspaper reporters were at the hospital waiting outside for an interview, but I quickly slipped out unnoticed. It was an honor to have cared for him.

Shreekant went on to train in plastic and reconstructive surgery and is now in private practice in Lakeland, Florida. Some years ago, Dr. Kumar brought him to our home one night as a surprise. When I opened the door all I could do was cry with joy. Dr. "Raju" Sivi Kumar is another pearl and then some. A few times during his residency we had slight disagreements, but he was always polite and "took it." He was an outstanding resident and then trained as a surgical intensivist at Upstate before returning as member of the surgical staff at St. Joseph's. He is an excellent technician.

When reflecting on Shreekant Tripathi and Raju Kumar it seems appropriate to narrate a fascinating case unusual then but, much more commonplace now in emergency rooms of Upstate and St. Joseph's.

It concerned D. S., a 24-year-old male brought to St. Joseph's emergency room at 4 a.m. in July 1980 with a stab wound to the left chest. He was in shock with evidence of cardiac tamponade. Tamponade is an external compression of the heart with a resultant inability for the heart to pump effectively. This is usually due to an accumulation of fluid within the pericardium or sac around the heart. Surprisingly, I was called in, although I had not performed heart surgery for eight years. The patient was cross matched for blood transfuse and rushed to the operating room, where Tripathi, Kumar and I performed a rapid left anterior thoracotomy. En route to the operating room blood was continually removed from the pericardial sac using an aspirating syringe.

The pericardial sac about the heart was tense with blood. This was incised and the blood evacuated. A laceration one inch in length was found in the left ventricle and immediately closed over the index finger with three sutures. Bleeding was well controlled, however, the blood loss had been excessive and in spite of eight units (four quarts of blood) cardiac arrest occurred. This resulted in cardiac manual massage for 25 minutes by the three of us. An additional laceration of the lung was found and repaired. The incision was closed and his post-op course was thereafter satisfactory.

I was so pleased to have two of my favorites involved and needed them badly. This is undoubtedly a case that the three of us will never forget!

During the last few years of my practice, Dr. Kumar really spoiled me by scrubbing with me. He became an excellent chest surgeon in addition to his other abilities. He now uses the DaVinci robot and may have been the first to use it at St. Joe's. I facetiously told him he was the "second best chest surgeon in Central New York" I have great affection and admiration for him.

Recently, Dr. Kumar told me that our patient, D. S., had reappeared several years ago in the emergency room with a gall bladder attack. He remembered Kumar from his emergency surgery and Kumar was able to confirm that the patient had a satisfactory result from his heart repair.

Dr. Richie Unger and I experienced a very interesting situation together that I will never forget. He was an excellent resident. I shall always remember the very first case of a thoracic outlet syndrome done at St. Joseph's in 1964. The patient had associated causalgia and was referred by my good friend Dr. Francis Caliva. I had never seen a patient with thoracic outlet syndrome (TOS) but, was familiar with it. Further the association of causalgia was fascinating.

Frank was a classmate of mine in the freshman year but had to sit out for one year because of illness. He went on to become a professor of medicine at Upstate, and in 1962, was appointed Medical Director and Director of the Family Practice Program at St. Joseph's. He was an outstanding person and physician who contributed greatly to the Family Physician's Program.

The thoracic outlet is a space between the collar bone (clavicle) and the first rib. Through this pass the subclavian artery and vein and brachial nerve plexus to the upper extremity. If this space is compromised symptoms referable to the arm ensue. Narrowing of the subclavian artery is associated with numbness, tingling, and pallor in the arm. Subclavian vein narrowing gives cyanosis, swelling, and tingling. Brachial plexus involvement produces weakness, numbness, and tingling depending on the specific nerve roots involved. Usually ulnar nerve irritation with numbness and tingling of the fourth and fifth fingers is present. Often, more than one condition may be present rather than TOS alone.

It is crucial to make the correct diagnosis and equally important to carry out the proper treatment. TOS is caused by mechanical reduction of the space and the only effective treatment is to enlarge the area, i.e. remove the ceiling (clavicle) or the floor (1st rib). Claviculectomy is a very disabling procedure and unsightly as well. First rib resection is the treatment of choice. This approach was familiar to the chest surgeons performing thoracoplasties in the past as it was done in the high back of the chest.

I had planned on this incision to perform both procedures. To my knowledge, surgical treatment for this condition had never been done in Syracuse. The day before the operation, surgical resident Richie Unger, who was scheduled to assist me, called very excited. He had just read an article in the latest *Annals of Surgery Journal* using a new surgical approach for TOS, namely transaxillary first rib resection by Dr. David Roos of Denver.

I later became friendly with Dr. Roos while visiting Denver. He popularized first-rib resections for TOS. The transaxillary first rib resection approach is ingenious. I call it the "Hollywood incision." However it is not to be taken lightly as the exposure is more limited. Experience and excellent assistance are absolute requisites.

After reading about the procedure, I agreed to use this approach. Any second thoughts were short lived. The first rib was resected and sympathectomy performed with no difficulty. I appreciated Dr. Unger's assistance because the exposure was much more difficult to obtain. The cosmetic result was worth it and the patient did very well.

Since then, I have performed hundreds of similar procedures, using this approach in all. Thank you, Richie!

Dr. Evan Dentes was an excellent surgical resident who rotated from Upstate to St. Joseph's.A fine physical specimen, he was always upbeat and energetic along with being respectful and dependable. He is a fine technician and remains one of my favorites.

Dr. Roy Buerkle, Jr. came to St. Joe's as a surgical resident prior to beginning his orthopedic training. He was always pleasant, dependable and a fine physician. I feel a close connection with him.

Dr. Roberto Canto, originally from Cuba, where his family experienced the treachery of Fidel Castro in his early years of deception, is very special to me. He came to St. Joseph's as a surgical resident for one year and then went into a urology residency. During that year we had a great association professionally and socially. I have found him to be extremely capable, reliable and intelligent. After returning to San Juan to take his residency and start private practice in urology, we have continued to remain in contact.

He and his wife Jossie have been so gracious and giving to us. Two years ago they insisted on our staying at their condo in the Dorado Beach area and entertained us all at their expense. No one has ever done this for me except my parents and brother. He has been very successful in his field of medicine in San Juan and recently built a lovely three story home with elevator on the golf course in the Dorado Beach area as their summer home. I am very proud of him.

We have great memories of visiting with the Cantos. Before departing on a Carribean Cruise out of San Juan, the Cantos picked us up at our hotel and insisted on taking us to Old San Juan and show us the sites. While sitting in an outside café eating ice cream, I entered the restaurant to use the men's room. The female owner refused the use of the facility. Dr. Canto shouted in Spanish, "do you know that's Dr. George Heitzman!"

Out of nowhere, a male voice had screamed out "Dr. Heitzman!" and came rushing towards me. It was Louie, a waiter there, and Dr. Barreto's stepfather. Can you imagine this happening in a Spanish-speaking city 2 million people? Needless to say I was allowed to use the bathroom!

Shortly thereafter, the Canto's insisted on taking us to a family christening. We were very hesitant on intruding and had no idea what to expect. It was a two-hour ride to the event being held at his cousin's country farm. His cousin was an engineer, and in addition became very successful in growing mangos and exporting them throughout the world. This so-called farm was actually an estate fully equipped with horses giving tours to the orchards.

The event was held outdoors, fully catered with multiple pig roasts on a spit. It was an elegant event under the sunset that ended with a spectacular firework display. We were treated like royalty. My wife enjoyed this very much and has always identified with their culture. We realize that the Cubans are a very important part of the Puerto Rican economy.

When I stopped performing surgery in 1988 I felt well in every respect, with the exception of noting subtle changes by the medical insurance companies. Previously, I could decide when to admit a patient for surgery with no problem. Most of my patients were old--some in their eighties--and they required a chest operation. This is formidable in any age group let alone the elderly. The majority had lung cancers and had recently stopped smoking at my insistence. It was imperative to prepare them for the most demanding medical procedure of their lifetime.

For that reason, I frequently admitted the poor risks and elderly one week before surgery. During this pre-operative time, intensive respiratory treatments were initiated, such as bronchodilators, to diminish spasm or constriction of the breathing tubes and to improve their overall stamina. I personally walked patients up and down three flights of stairs daily to be satisfied they could withstand the surgery and immediate post-operative period. I frankly cannot recall how this was initiated, but it worked like a charm!

I found this routine extremely effective and a very high percentage of these patients tolerated their lung resections very well and improved markedly. There were very few failures, primarily those who could not improve significantly in order to proceed with surgery.

At the time of my retirement, it became necessary to

obtain permission from the insurance company for this "early pre-operative admission," and it became more and more difficult to do so. Increasing similar restrictions emerged and the main thrust appeared to be to reduce hospital costs more than to obtain good patient outcomes.

It is important to remember that this was before the advent of performing chest procedures via the much better tolerated mini incisions. I had never envisioned admitting octogenarians for major chest procedures the day of the surgery and am still appalled it is done. Incredibly, with the smaller incisions and less traumatic surgery most patients survive.

Undoubtedly, much more morbidity occurs than is reported. Several years ago, a close friend in whom I had removed a lung cancer with long term survival had a redo coronary bypass. He was discharged after a brief post-operative stay with marked swelling of his legs and heart failure. He had been given no specific orders.

Another patient's wife had a similar bypass procedure and went home a few days after surgery with a significant collection of chest fluid unrecognized and untreated.

It is very difficult for me to accept the current standards as advantageous to the patient.

Shortly after retiring from surgery, I took a position

examining patients' hospital charts for a medical group, the Peer Review Organization (PRO). This was formed under a federal bureaucracy firmly entrenched in Washington D.C. for many years, the Health Care Finance Administration (HCFA). Its purpose allegedly is to examine patient's charts to evaluate the quality of care given by their physicians. As I worked there, I realized that my fellow physicians had no idea of the workings of HFCA and the newly created PRO.

Dr. Richard "Buzz" Eberle has been a long-standing friend. He was an excellent surgeon and also had a very intense interest in the New York State Medical Society have been a past president at the county and state level. He was the leader in the Syracuse PRO and an excellent one. Buzz was tuned in on the medical political process and made frequent visits to the medical society headquarters in Lake Success, New York. He and I made several trips to the local county medical society meetings to enlighten the members on the workings of the PRO.

Until then, very few had any awareness of the system, which included penalizing physicians for relatively simple situations that they were totally ignorant of. It became more apparent to me that this bureaucracy was a police of medicine with very little worthiness. It had been thrust upon doctors with little or no preparation or warning. I learned that the medical society's contract with HFCA was an annual and was shortly up for renewal. When I asked for more information, I was assured that there was no concern from the New York State Medical Society. Nonetheless, on the renewal date the contract was awarded to a subsidiary medical society of Long Island, actually a member of our New York State Society!

Again, I realized how little I knew about medical politics. Needless to say I resigned from the PRO, bewildered. and am still shaking my head.

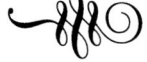

Chapter Seventeen

ART

Both brother Jim and I had some degree of talent in drawing dating back to grammar and high school. He had an amazing ability to sketch people in action, an indication of his wonderful imagination. However, he always made little of the talent and almost hid it. I cannot recall that he even took art courses in high school. I took mechanical drawing and other art, but I never was "the artist".

In medical school, Jim and I both excelled in parasitology because we could draw. I feel that the most outstanding teacher in medical school was Justus Mueller, PhD. He was undoubtedly a genius in many fields. He was editor of the prestigious *Journal of Parasitology* and owned a company that manufactured models of various parasites with their life cycles. He frequently made trips to the Amazon to perform original experiments. In Dr. Mueller's class, being able to draw and sketch placed you in a very special group. Both Jim and I qualified much to the disgust of our buddies who were not so endowed.

As president of our class, I had the occasion to know Dr. Mueller in a greater capacity, as each class presented a portrait of a faculty member as a donation to the medical school.

Justus was an excellent artist himself and a close friend of the best portrait artist in Central New York, Joe Kozlowski. I had the privilege of meeting Joe at the time we commissioned him to do a portrait of Dr. E.C. Reifenstein, Professor of Medicine. This painting was outstanding and hangs today in the medical school.

There was a hiatus of many years before my relationship with Joe was renewed. That was in the early sixties when I contacted him to take art lessons, which became one of the highlights of my life.

I started working with charcoal to develop values. After this, he introduced me to oils, acrylics and pastels. Learning this was so important to me, especially in the early seventies when life was grim. After a short time, Joe would not accept any remuneration. He proved to become one of my very best friends, as was his wife, Mary. Both were brilliant in different ways and I learned so much from them. Mary was an expert with investments. I found many years ago never to play scrabble with them. It was so embarrassing!

For the past 20 years, I have continued to paint, mainly with water colors and occasionally with pastels. My oldest and dearest friend, since grammar school, Bob Peet and I started painting together. Our weekly meetings consisted of painting and then lunch. It was a wonderful camaraderie until his death in 2009.

Bob was a much better artist than I in high school and before enlisting for World War II he had planned to be a commercial artist. Instead, he ended up with an excellent position with the New York Telephone Company.

Joe offered to do my portrait in 1978 and it is one of my prize possessions. He included in the background one of my favorite, personal watercolors. The portrait hangs in our den. I am flattered that he always looked at me as a fellow artist rather than a surgeon.

Joe has done many portraits of the faculty members of the Upstate College of Medicine. There have been a very few portraits done by others. The difference is striking in that Joe's work is so much superior. One of the quickest ways of identifying a portrait artist's ability is to observe the subject's hands. Less capable artists conceal the hands by hiding them in pockets or behind the body. Unfortunately, others show the hands.

Painting is my passion, and like medicine, cannot be totally captured. Art has always been a great "medicine" for me. I can recall painting into the late hours and becoming so engrossed that I lost track of time. It would be 3 a.m. with scheduled surgery only hours away. Yet it was so medicinal and counteracted difficult times in my life.

Perhaps one of my best works is a pastel of a champion trotter, a French horse, Sophora, owned by our dear friends, the late Jane and Nick Colella. They were horse owners and very active at Vernon Downs when it was a famous track. Unfortunately this champion died in a barn fire and this was devastating to them. They cherished a small photograph of the horse. Using this as a guide, I did a large pastel of Sophora and presented it to them in the late 1970s. Nick and Jane were so appreciative of this gift, it hung next to their original Rubens in their home filled with priceless art and antiques. Some 30 years later, Jane passed away and Nick, also ill, personally delivered it to our home, where it hangs in the family room today.

Gina and I have enjoyed art together. She prefers to visit the sights of the greats, preferably Italy and France. Italy is by far our favorite country to visit where we began 30 years ago on our honeymoon. Although I could go on and on to discuss my love for the food, culture and architecture the subject will be limited to art.

In Rome we have spent hours absorbing the overwhelming beauty of Michelangelo's paintings on the ceiling of the Sistine Chapel and his sculpture of the Pieta that sits in the magnificent St. Peter's Basilica.

Florence is considered the art and cultural center of Italy. The Cathedral of Santa Maria del Fiore (Duomo) is the crowning glory of Florence. Its multi colored pastel marble exterior is breathtaking. Florence is the home of Michelangelo and his famous David in the Galleria dell'Accademia.. It is also the home of many of Leonardo DaVinci's masterpieces that sit in the Galleria degli Uffizi. Michelangelo is buried in the Basilica di Santa Croce in Florence. It is incredible indeed that two of the world's greatest geniuses lived in the same locale at the same time.

We have appreciated the beauty and art of Capri, Sorrento and Sicily's Taormina.

In 1994, Gina and I visited France and stayed in Paris. Our favorite artists are the impressionists, Monet and Renoir. Museum D'Orsay contained the majority of their works. The Louvre houses the famous Mona Lisa by Leonardo DaVinci as well as Rodin's sculptor of The Thinker. The Cathedral of Notre Dame is a beautiful structure indeed. Another highlight was traveling to Giverny, Monet's home. We visited in June and the gardens were at their peak with rambling rose bushes and of course the famous water lilies.

Versaille is an incredible architectural palace with formal gardens and rich history. On a Mediterranean cruise we visited Barcelona, Spain.We enjoyed Gaudi's architecture including the Sagrado Familia Cathedral. Monaco in the French Riviera is filled with tremendous beauty and art.

In London, England we visited the famous St. Thomas

Hospital, the home of Dr. James Cyriax and professor in orthopedic medicine. I visited the center and observed their method of manipulation and massage and its application to cervical strains. I saw this as a tool in the treatment of patients who were referred to me as having thoracic outlet syndrome but, in reality had neck problems, cervical strains.

My two loves interchangeably, are medicine and art. They have sustained me.

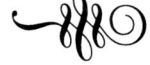

Chapter Eighteen

MY BROTHER

Readers will note that the subject my brother, Jim, frequently surfaces in this book. This is inevitable as he has been so important in my life from childhood on. He always worked behind the scenes as he was always humble and quiet. However, those who knew him well will recall his ready smile and dry humor. As my mother frequently used to say "isn't he witty?"

Jim was extremely well liked by almost everyone, a regular guy who was down to earth. He knew all of the workers at St. Joseph's Hospital (electricians, painters, and plumbers) by their first names and had breakfast with them almost daily at the hospital. You can see why he was current on all hospital activities!

Jim did many generous things for people, mainly the underprivileged, and never talked about it. I am the sole person who knew of the many things he did for the house staff through the years at St. Joseph's. It was not at all uncommon for him to take an intern at the end of his tenure to a fine clothing store, such as the late Wells & Coverly, and buy him a suit or to the famous Nettleton Shoe Company, for a pair of world-famous shoes. This was always done without fanfare.

I do believe that Jim was very proud of my initiating open heart surgery in Syracuse and did everything possible to make that a reality at St. Joseph's Hospital in 1958. He was a huge contributor to the program but stayed behind the scenes.

It was very heartening to know that in a small way he was honored by the St. Joseph's Hospital Medical Staff on Friday, September 25, 1964, with a beautiful plaque: "In appreciation of and recognition for the devotion and scientific dedication in the organization of the Annual Cardiopulmonary Teaching Days 1958-1963." This is one of the few instances in his life where he was credited for every one to see. He was a most unusual individual in every respect and I am so proud of him. I have been miscredited many times for the many wonderful deeds he was in fact responsible for.

These annual cardiopulmonary teaching days he organized were extremely popular in the Syracuse medical community. They were held at the Syracuse Hotel and sponsored by St. Joseph's Hospital. Many world and nationally known physicians came as participants, including the best known cardiovascular and thoracic surgeon in the world, Dr. Michael DeBakey.

I shall never forget that at that meeting when Dr. Josh Malgieri approached Dr. DeBakey and introduced himself, saying he usually performed 100 or more vascular operations a year.

This immediately caught DeBakey's attention, and then Josh added, "Yes, I do. Hemorrhoidectomies!"

Dr. DeBakey was speechless as Josh laughed at his "joke." I was mortified.

My brother and I are credited on two medical papers "we" submitted for publication. One was "Myocardial Infarction Following Penetrating Wounds of the Heart," which appeared in *The American Journal of Cardiology,* 1960." The other was "Heitzman, Heitzman and Elliott: Primary Esophageal Amyloidosis" in the *Archives of Internal Medicine*, 1962." (Dr. Chuck Elliott was the third contributor. He was a house officer at St. Joe's at the time and later entered private practice in Fayetteville, New York.) Needless to say, Jim wrote both of them and they were excellent. My involvement was only with the surgery.

The case of amyloidosis was fascinating. This elderly patient was worked up and felt to have a cancer of the esophagus. Preoperatively a definite diagnosis was not made. Even at surgery frozen section of the mass to be removed was called cancer. Treatment consisted of a partial removal of the stomach and esophagus. Permanent sections revealed this lesion to be amyloidosis, a non-malignant lesion of unknown cause. This entity frequently involves several organs such as the kidneys, usually progresses and is fatal. However, the process did not progress in this patient in his 70s and he survived several years.

Dr. Jim's passion was fishing on Oneida Lake. As mentioned earlier, we spent our childhood summers there. He later inherited the cottage because of his intense love and appreciation for the place and continued to enjoy the area tremendously. He became an avid bass fisherman and learned many "spots" from Dr. Paul Cramer, a legendary hunter and fisherman.

It was truly an honor fishing with these two. Jim was a fine athlete who always enjoyed competition. This came from our Dad. As a youngster he was the head of the gang and played rough. As he grew up, this spirit was well controlled. He took up karate in mid-life and earned a black belt. He used to sleep with a sweat shirt on to hide his bruises from his wife, B.C. He also used to keep his weights under the bed and used them daily. He was quite a guy.

Jim and B.C. had five children: E. James Heitzman Jr., Ph.D, Mark Heitzman, M.D., Kristina Carr, P.A., Karen Heitzman, M.D., and Eric Heitzman, PhD.

Jim and BC had a wonderful marriage and traveled extensively throughout the world including Mexico, England, Europe, Russia to name a few. They also traveled on the Queen Elizabeth 2 and Concord. They went on safari expeditions in Africa and shared wonderful stories.

Sadly, Jim, Jr. passed away on November 15, 2008, at Stanford University Medical Center, from acute myeloid leukemia while awaiting a bone marrow transplant. He authored several books and papers about ancient and modern India.

Barbara, Brenna's and Ian's mother, has always been a great friend of B.C. and continues to be available and supportive to her even today.

The long weekend of June 28 and 29, 2009, was extremely meaningful. The cottage where our Aunts Frankie Hughes and Kate Drum had cared for Jim and me all those wonderful summers was to house a most important event.

Throughout our lives it had served as a very special haven for social gatherings but this pretty much ended with Jim's death in 1996.

During routine hernia surgery, a tumor was discovered and removed from Jim's scrotal area. It was a very rare malignant mesothelioma, a tumor more commonly found on the chest that is often related to asbestos exposure. Within a few months, Jim was gone. It's a loss from which I have never fully recovered.

Although his immediate family continued to spend many good times at the lake, this had lessened appreciably as most of his grown children were now living out of town or out of state. Jim's widow, B.C., was not well and had already sold the next door camp because of lack of use.

Jim, Jr. had been teaching the history of India in California. Disaster came when this splendid, big, bright, muscular fellow was stricken with leukemia. Initially, this was a more subtle bone marrow abnormality of unknown cause and responded fairly well to blood transfusions and a new drug. The last year, his condition worsened swiftly and a definite diagnosis of leukemia was made. He rapidly deteriorated and died at Stanford Medical Center with his siblings, Mark and Karen, as well as his children Brenna, and Ian, and his loyal wife Smriti, at his side. Their infant daughter Maitreyi was also in proximity. His sister Kristina had visited recently.

Jim, Jr. had converted to Hinduism and requested that his cremated ashes be spread on Oneida Lake. Preparations for this were made for the June weekend. Kristina and her siblings were in charge of this event. Also in attendance were their families and friends, as well as my own children from my first marriage, George Jr., Donna, Peter, and Jennifer along with their families, and my wife, Gina and our son Jacob. At 2 p.m., a boat with Smriti, Brenna, Ian, Mark and Kristina motored out with Jim's ashes, which were spread along with flowers in an area beyond Shackleton's Point. The remaining guests lined up by the dock in silence and waited for their return. This happening was truly beautiful in all respects.

Any differences in the past disappeared and were replaced with an aura of love, friendship, and tranquility. Goodwill prevailed over this gathering of more than 40 people. This is exactly what nephew Jim wanted on his memorial.

Earlier my son Peter had invited me to go fishing with him and his cousin Mark the next day. Mark is a physician and talented artist, while Pete is a professional guitarist.

Mark and Pete were very interested in fishing the famous spot where Uncle Joe Shebo had taken Jim and me years earlier, and this put considerable pressure on me. The three of us set out in a small aluminum boat, and they supplied all the fishing supplies. Fortunately, Gina had provided great lunches for us and I felt this would save me should our trip be unproductive.

We set out and headed for that area the other side of Shackleton's Point. That infamous fishing triumph had been more than 50 years ago and I was a bit apprehensive. As expected, we caught nothing in the "old spot" but we were very successful by working over the adjacent water and drifting. Interestingly, Peter was casting with trout lures and that proved the key to a very successful trip. Mark shortly followed suit. Yours truly caught absolutely nothing but the other two hauled in six beautiful black bass. Waiting for us at the camp were Smriti, Maitreyi and Ian.

We decided to follow tradition and fillet the fish. The six of us enjoyed a superb meal at the lake, providing a perfect ending to cap off a very special weekend.

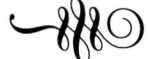

Chapter Nineteen

A ROLE REVERSAL

While Gina was driving me home from Crouse Memorial Hospital in October, 2008, we began discussing this memoir when she quipped, "You have to include these last few days and share your changing role."

Dr. Jim Longo and his associates have been my cardiologists for several years and, together with internist Dr. Dick Hehir, I have felt very secure.

On the eve of October 8, while preparing for bed, I sensed an irregular heart rate. It was atrial fibrillation, a condition where the two reservoirs of the heart rapidly beat 200 or more per minute. These rates are in part conducted to the two pumps or ventricles, usually 120 to 130 beats per minute. This heart rate is well tolerated for considerable time unless other cardiac problems are also present. I was totally asymptomatic.

The most serious drawback with atrial fibrillation is that such a rapid atrial rate over more than 24 hours can lead to clotting of the blood in the atrium with possible clots breaking off to other body parts, including the brain with stroke. Therefore there is a relatively safe window.

At 1 a.m., I spoke with one of Jim's partners, who advised going to the Crouse emergency room. He would leave orders. When Gina and I arrived, the atrial fibrillation spontaneously stopped and converted to a normal rhythm. I was checked out thoroughly and observed for approximately one more hour. I had been totally without symptoms throughout and had I not been familiar with the condition, it could easily have gone unrecognized.

In talking with Dr. Longo the next day, he indicated atrial fibrillation (AF) usually spontaneously subsides although it often recurs. He advised, should it happen again, to wait several hours before going to the emergency room.

I felt perfectly fine performing the usual activities including exercise until 7 p.m. four days later, when a rapid irregular heart rate recurred. I slept through the night but, on awakening the next morning, the condition was still present. I remained totally asymptomatic. We called Longo's office and were advised to come right in. When he examined me, the E.K.G. showed a very fast irregular rate due to atrial flutter rather than atrial fibrillation. He said that this was an easier condition to treat but if left untreated the results were similar to atrial fibrillation, including clots in the left atrium.

We were taken to the cardiac care floor of Crouse Hospital. After ascertaining that I had not eaten for several hours and aspiration of stomach contents had been excluded, I was given an intravenous anesthetic and electrocardioverted with a single shock. The result was a slower heart rate but not a normal sinus rhythm. As this was relatively unstable and could revert to other arrhythmias, a permanent pacemaker was advised.

This took me by complete surprise. I had inserted the first cardiac pacemaker in Syracuse 47 years earlier at St. Joseph's Hospital. Between then and my retirement in 1988, I inserted many, many units and witnessed amazingly rapid improvements in their approach, function, and design.

As described earlier, the first pacemaker insertion required an open left chest incision with suturing two electrodes to the surface of the chief heart pump, the left ventricle. This was a "big" procedure, as one is almost always operating on an older age group in their 70s, 80s, and older.

The oldest patient I personally operated on was 100 years old but, fortunately, this was some years later when the simpler transvenous approach was available.

The principle of the current technique was introduced in the 1960s and revolutionized the procedure in every respect. For the past 40 years, the approach consists of using local anesthesia with a "light' intravenous medication to produce amnesia. The incision is usually below the left clavicle (collar bone) and a small pocket is made in the subcutaneous tissue. Under fluoroscopy one or two wires (electrodes) are inserted into an adjacent vein and threaded into the right chambers of the heart. Originally only one was placed into the right ventricle and both left and right pumps were stimulated. In time, two wires were used, one in the right ventricle and the other in the right atrium. The two wires stimulated first the atria and then the ventricles, producing a more normal sequence of first atrial and then ventricular pacing.

Amazing strides were also made in reducing battery size while vastly increasing its function. Currently, the battery size is approximately that of a silver dollar and several times its thickness. Some pacemaker generators are capable of detecting the usual fatal ventricular tachycardias and ventricular fibrillation and automatically cardiovert the heart to a normal sinus rhythm.

The tremendous revolutionary changes in the development of cardiac pacemakers rank extremely high in improvements in medicine in my life time.

When my rapid irregular heart rate occurred I had no thoughts whatever of having a pacemaker inserted! Two of Dr. Longo's partners perform the pacemaker implantations. They are board certified cardiologists who have acquired the additional surgical expertise of inserting pacemakers. The strong advantage of this is that they are familiar with all aspects of cardiology including their expertise interpreting the key of this procedure the electrocardiogram.

Dr. Anthony Navone implanted my Medtronic dual chamber pacemaker without incident. Before anesthesia, I met him and found him to be delightful in every way and he gained my confidence. The procedure went very smoothly and my postoperative course was very uneventful. Gina consulted with the operating room nurse and Dr. Navone, along with anesthesiologist, and it was decided that I would be very-well sedated for fear that I would take over the procedure!

The operating room staff was extremely supportive in every way, as was the hospital staff that evening and the following day. Somehow they understood the difficulty that I was experiencing in this reversed role as a patient and allowed me to be part of the team in the decision-making process.

Needless to say, Dr. Jim Longo was present throughout and cared for me in a fine manner. A checkup in his office on the seventh post-op day revealed excellent progress in every respect.

There are very few precautions to follow. Cell phones should not be held within six inches from the pacemaker. In airports, metal detectors should be avoided as pacemakers may set off an alarm. The security officer may use a wand or does a hand search instead. Security metal detectors will not harm the pacemaker.

A note of interest: As a physician, I have been familiar with the Medtronic pacemaker and its company for many years and used its products often... It is by far one of the most outstanding pacemaker companies in the world. I personally visited the company headquarters in Minneapolis, Minnesota, and was treated in a very fine manner.

The procedure had a considerable psychological affect on me for many reasons, and as my wife has said, I undoubtedly am in a more secure position now than I have been for quite some time. In addition I can appreciate even more what I have always maintained, "I would rather take care of patients any day rather than be one."

The subject of pacemakers provides an opportune time to discuss one of the many changes in medicine. There are countless changes now as never before. The term "interventionalist" is appearing more frequently, particularly in regards to thoracic surgery and its effect on the future of the chest surgeon. I define the interventionalist as a board-certified specialist in his/her field including cardiology, radiology, gastroenterology, and pulmonary medicine who performs or participates in surgically related procedures.

When performing chest surgery in the 1980s until retiring, I noted an occasional situation where a medical colleague professed a desire to perform a procedure heretofore assumed exclusively to the role of the surgeon.

These requests were quite rare and more or less ignored. I have always felt that the doctor performing a procedure should be personally capable of taking care of any untoward incidence or complication relating to it; otherwise he should never attempt it.

With passage of time, obviously there were more and more non surgeons who disagree with this philosophy and proceeded to instrument patients, usually without incident. Should complications occur, they call in the thoracic surgeon to deal with the problem. I recall more than one case of a foreign-body lodged in the esophagus, such as a bone, piece of meat, or a coin where the medical specialist was unable to remove it after multiple attempts. On one occasion serious damage was done with perforation of the esophagus. I was called in to perform an emergency chest operation with repair of the esophagus and removal of the foreign body. Coincidentally, most often I was called in on a sunny Saturday afternoon while fishing on Oneida Lake with brother Jim.

I personally did not experience the radiologists who drain chest abscesses or needle biopsy lung lesions with complications as they did not perform such when I was practicing.

The implanting of pacemakers I feel is different. The original pacemakers were inserted via a thoracotomy, and without question the chest surgeon performed the procedure. In a very short time, however, the majority of operations were done via the transvenous route and the generators became much more sophisticated and more useful. Only the cardiologists were knowledgeable enough to thoroughly understand and evaluate what generators were needed and how they performed. Understandably, they became the implanters of such highly technical equipment. The surgical incisions themselves were relatively simple.

Although many current heart specialists prefer to practice pure medical cardiology alone, the field includes a great deal of instrumentation and many cardiologists are involved with heart catheterizations, angioplasties, and placement of stents. They have become much more surgery-oriented.

Revolutionary changes are occurring in the field of thoracic and cardiovascular surgery. Not only are cardiac procedures changing with smaller less-invasive operations utilizing the robot, etc., in its infancy, aortic valve replacement is being done with a team of interventionalist cardiologists, radiologists, and heart surgeons. The valve is introduced via the femoral artery and guided into position in the heart under fluoroscopy without any chest incisions whatever. This is one of many factors in reducing thoracic surgical residencies by one third, truly a significant statistic.

Progressively, more thoracic operations, both cardiac and non cardiac, are being done without thoracic incisions. It would seem reasonable, however, to believe that fundamental knowledge and experience with the "old" incisions should be a requisite, should unforeseen complications arise.

We have a new "breed" of doctors in hospitals today. The term "ist" is being used more and more and is another indicator of the changes in the practice of medicine. With this there is further diminution of private practice and concomitant use of hospital-salaried physicians.

Doctors who work for and exclusively in hospitals are called "hospitalists" and first appeared in the 1990s. They care for hospital patients where their own physicians are overworked with their office practices or prefer not to engage in hospital care. "Hospitalist" was a common name but, now there are wide varieties of "ists." One of the original "ists" was the intensivist, who cares for intensive care patients and who has a very demanding job. In time, many other varieties have appeared. "Proceduralists" perform one or more specialized activities repeatedly; "interventionalists" perform heart-related angioplasties and stent insertions. More recently "nocturnists" have appeared and carry out emergency surgical care overnight.

Theoretically, this provides a more efficient and profitable way to run a business.

I muse whether they would be willing to walk my patients up and down stairs in preparation for surgery? Will the next "ist" be the "walkerist?"

Chapter Twenty

VITAMINS AND NUTRITION

Despite my recent cardiac events, I have enjoyed a long and healthy life. While I certainly do not claim to have "all the answers" on any subject, I am a true believer in preventive health and nutrition.

First of all, neither Jim nor I ever smoked. Our father was a long-standing heavy cigarette smoker until we pressured him into stopping when he was in his sixties. Thereafter, he used to keep an unlit cigar in his mouth but never smoked. We always played high school sports and felt athletics and smoking did not mix. We never used tobacco throughout our lives.

During World War II, the nicest gift to send to troops overseas was considered a carton of cigarettes; I am convinced that this was a significant factor in the great increase in smoking in the 1940s. Unquestionably, this led to the progressive increased incidence of lung cancer, which for many years has been the number-one cancer killer in men and number two for women.

My medical practice was dependant on the popular use of tobacco. There is no question in my mind that smoking tobacco is directly related to almost all lung cancers in both sexes. In addition, it is a causative factor in coronary artery disease.

I truly believe that without tobacco the need for chest surgeons in Central New York would be reduced to a handful. Currently, there are at least one dozen in the Syracuse-area alone.

Antioxidants are substances that combat oxidants, materials that cause debilitating conditions such as cancer and arteriosclerosis . For decades, the world famous physicist Lynus Pauling had advocated large doses of vitamin C (ascorbic acid) daily and claimed benefits in promoting health. I, too, have used large doses of all water-soluble vitamins (vitamins B & C) as they are not retained and are rapidly excreted. This is not the case of fat-soluble vitamins (vitamins A, D,E,& K) as they are absorbed and stored in the body. Fat-soluble vitamin toxicity is widely recognized. By using these vitamins for many years along with daily exercise (treadmill, sit-ups, push-ups, and weight lifting), I have felt well and have been very fortunate to enjoy good health. While, I cannot prove that they work, I think they do. Why change?

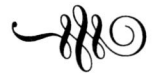

Chapter Twenty One

REFLECTIONS ON A LIFE IN MEDICINE

What can the current medical student or young physician gain from my experience? That is very difficult to answer in view of the many years ago that I was a medical student and then a cardiovascular thoracic surgeon in private practice.

So many changes have taken place the last 50 years that medical students' and young physicians' lives then and now are drastically different.

When Jim and I were medical students from 1944-47, the average class had 40-some students, including only two or three females. The selection process was less standardized and unquestionably a doctor's son or daughter was favored to be admitted. The effect of World War II definitely was a big factor. With few exceptions, the rapport between faculty and students was often unfriendly and antagonistic.

As president of our class, I had more familiarity with the faculty including the dean, but I never felt I ever accomplished a great deal or had any rapport with him. The class mortality was nearly a third, and many students were failed without any notice. There appeared to be no incentive or desire to warn students who were not doing satisfactorily or any attempt to help them. To be sure there were exceptions to this attitude. The person who stands out even after these many years was pediatrician Dr. Bill Kopel. He was an excellent teacher and a true friend of the students.

In both pre-med and medical school my friends and I had a real fear of failure. It would have been very embarrassing to us and our families not to succeed. We had pride. These feelings carried on through internship and residency training. Admittedly, competition was also an extremely strong factor. This began in pre-med and actually has never ended. Training positions were relatively few and one's work ethic was a key.

Behind all this was the family, our parents and close relatives and friends. The family unit was extremely strong and paramount. We medical students were expected to excel and make our families proud of us. Our parents were very supportive. Loans were unheard of. I could never have pursued eight years of internship and residency with no or a paltry salary without my parent's financial help.

Terms "right" and "wrong" were frequently used and recognized. "God" had significant meaning.

Gradually, significant changes have occurred to a point where what I have described is unknown or treated with contempt and disgust. It would appear that a very large number of high school and college students have a much different orientation. Materialism abounds while achievement and self drive have appreciatively lessened. Thoughts of the future are measured in months and not beyond four years. "Now" is the driving force; instant gratification is the goal. The words "right" and "wrong" are almost obsolete and God is now spelled god.

I am the first to admit there are exceptions, thank the Lord.

These are exciting times in medicine irrespective of persistent drawbacks such as the crippling effects of a savage federal bureaucracy, the Health Care Finance Agency (HCFA) that began making it very difficult for physicians as early as the 1990s or sooner. The only politician I ever heard mention HCFA and the need to replace or change it was Newt Gingrich, on a single occasion when he was speaker of the House of Representatives. Another tremendous drawback to medicine is the trial malpractice lawyers with their powerful lobby in Washington, DC. The current medical malpractice suits are largely responsible for the outrageous medical malpractice insurance. For this reason, many capable healthy physicians are retiring early as some have to pay over $125,000.00 annually for medical malpractice insurance.

Embarrassingly, there are members of our medical profession who travel throughout the state making a living testifying for malpractice lawyers. Some are not even board certified in the medical specialty they are testifying about. Nonetheless, they are paid handsomely for their medical "expertise."

Health insurance premiums are unduly exorbitant for several reasons. One is the high cost to run the health insurance companies. Last year, our local newspaper reported that four top executives in my health insurance company were each receiving well over one million dollars annually. Isn't there something wrong here?

While the pharmacist has always been an extremely important factor in medicine, he/she has had a much more significant role for the last two decades as health insurance companies have a larger voice in the medications prescribed to patients.

From the time I graduated from medical school over 60 years ago, few if any doctors had a complete grasp of pharmaceuticals, as their numbers were voluminous even then. It was common place to consult the pharmacist frequently concerning drugs and their specifics. The physician always wrote the prescription, including dose and particular orders, but additional advice from the druggist was most helpful.

Over time, the drug industry has become a huge multibillion-dollar industry. The medications now available, and their specific uses, challenge both the pharmacist and physician. The new generic products available during the past year alone are incredible even in my own personal experience. Some of my prescriptions are replaced by new generics several times a year with a rationale by the insurance company of keeping prices down. Excellent rapport between the medical and pharmaceutical professions is an absolute must for the nation's health.

Several years ago I had the privilege of seeing endocrinologist Dr. Mickey Lebowitz for a non-serious thyroid condition. I soon realized how special and thorough he was, a truly outstanding physician in many ways. It was indeed a surprise to later learn that he had given up his very busy private practice and never knew the circumstances until reading his exceptionally well-crafted book *Losing My Patience: Why I Quit The Medical Game.*

Gina and I read about a book-signing in the newspaper and were two of many attendees of this event at the local Barnes and Noble. As usual he was very attentive.

His book is extremely well done in many respects and illustrates in splendid fashion why he was obliged to stop the private practice of medicine. He provides considerable objective and subjective data to support his feelings that to practice good private medicine is next to impossible in the United States. I began reading the book on vacation and found I could not put it down; it was so well done and came straight from the heart.

Mickey graduated from medical school in 1988 and started private practice in 1991. Interestingly I retired in 1988 for similar reasons. He illustrates in considerable detail the insurmountable and impossible hurdles to take proper care of his patients because of escalating malpractice insurance premiums as engineered by trial lawyers with their powerful lobby. Horrendous drug prescription costs force many patients who can't afford them to choose between their medications or food.

Without adequate medication, many patients cannot be properly treated, with ensuing poor results and frustrated physicians. The excessive premiums for health insurance companies increase annually while insurance executives command salary increases. My health insurance company pays three executives each well in excess of $1 million annually; one receives almost $2 million.

With the poor insurance reimbursement rates (which are progressively decreasing) Mickey was not able to sustain his high level of care or his very modest life style. He was not willing to run a factory-operated assembly line. He could not live with himself. I could not either. In the end we see excellent doctors exit the field much sooner than expected and others choosing alternate careers rather than medicine.

In earlier years a doctor would dream that one or more

of his children would follow his or her footsteps and choose the field of medicine. Currently, it is very common to hear doctors say that they are happy that their children have not chosen medicine as a career and they do not encourage them to do so.

The chief reason that I retired was because of the increasing control and limitations on physicians by health insurance companies. As an illustration, many of my patients in need of chest surgery were in their seventies and eighties with lung cancer. In those times, small incisions and newer techniques with less extensive procedures and less debility had not yet been developed.

Major lung surgery for lung resection required a large chest incision and was associated with a marked degree of pain and debility postoperatively in all age groups. I found that in order to prepare these elderly patients for major surgery that they had to be in top physical condition. Therefore they were admitted to the hospital for one or more weeks in preparation. During this period I would personally walk up and down two to three flights of stairs to prepare them for a post operative stressful recovery. If they were unable to perform this program it was obvious that surgery was contraindicated because they could not tolerate such. Amazingly most of these individuals responded well to this preparation and progressed satisfactorily during and after surgery. Very few were turned down.

As time passed I received more and more calls from insurance companies refusing early admissions. These calls I personally handled were from young people employed with little or no knowledge about the subject. I became aware of the course of events and realized that soon I could no longer be approved or successful in my preoperative plans. I was not willing to conform. I refused to admit my patient the morning of scheduled chest surgery knowing the outcome without proper preparation would likely be poor. One could have a lengthy discussion on what the cost would be to the taxpayer for this poor result. My primary interest was a good result for my patient.

This was happening for approximately two to three years before I retired and was a sampling of what Dr. Lebowitz experienced when he began practice and the ensuing twenty plus years. His book is highly recommended for all.

As I write about this topic President Barack Obama signed into law a highly controversial health care reform contrary to public opinion and the support of even one Republican congressman. It is alarming to witness the anger and violence directed toward the proponents.

My personal opinion is that if this health care reform remains in effect the quality of medicine will deteriorate.

There will be fewer applicants to medical school with a shortage of doctors in practice to care for an increasing patient population. The burdening tax structure to pay for this plan is astronomical and will be with us for decades.

I recall having been in practice a few years before the passage of Medicaid in the 1960s. Prior to this all doctors cared for patients irrespective of financial status. All patients were treated as needed and no one was turned down. Again, our liberal politicians passed the Medicaid law to cover almost all those without insurance in order for everyone "to be able to have his or her own doctor." In other words, "Entitlement!" Now, I was forced to give health care to more people at a personal cost to me to sustain this system.

This was not supported by most physicians because it was realized that the tremendous cost was unsustainable. The country is aware of our financial burden of the three entitlements: Social Security, Medicare and Medicaid. I do believe most Americans wish to support and sustain Social Security and Medicare to help our elderly. These are tremendous financial burdens to our country. Adding Medicaid has created an almost impossible challenge. Many people are aware of the tremendous abuses of this entitlement and how it can be negatively enabling. Medicaid was passed into law by a very liberal political party and the same is happening today with health care reform. It has become so unpopular that most physicians will no longer care for Medicaid patients because there is no profit in this whatsoever and the paperwork is so excessive.

The health care proposal recently signed into law by the president and passed in Congress without public and Republican support is another example of forcing changes on us. The result again is creation of many more problems along with much higher taxes. Do any of us understand what one trillion dollars is and what a tax of many, many trillion will mean to our children, grandchildren and great grandchildren?

Despite the very real problems with the business and politics of medicine, the current innovations in practice truly blow my mind. Aortic heart valves are now beginning to be replaced via an artery in the groin and then directed into the aorta to the heart valve site using fluoroscopy. Heart surgeons are now accompanied by the cardiologists and radiologists, now called "interventionists." It will be interesting to note how harmoniously this arrangement will work. One can visualize the revolutionary changes taking place; including how specifically these teams of doctors will be trained and integrated. Incidentally, one third of residency training spots in thoracic surgery are not filled at this time.

Such procedures and even more like them will be limited to large medical centers for financial reasons. There will be no place for the thoracic surgeon in private practice.

Another mind-boggling event is the injection of immature heart cells into the area of the recent heart attack (myocardial infarction) to replace the dead heart muscle and restore viable heart muscle and cardiac function. This is done by heart catheterization, a procedure many decades in existence. What other brilliant concepts have yet to come to fruition?

When I was a medical student, and until fairly recently, most physicians in training had no idea specifically what field we wished to follow: surgery, medicine, family practice, etc. It was not until we had graduated and began working in hospitals as interns that we decided specifically what we wanted. The reasoning was that we did not have the experience from our limited clinical training in school to enable our choosing specifically what field to follow.

The year of internship exposed us to the many various fields, allowing us to make a reasonable, informed decision about what course to choose as a career.

Currently, the fourth-year medical student must determine what field he or she wishes to follow, including specialties and sub-specialties. The student is accepted into this specific training program or residency immediately after graduation from medical school. I am truly amazed that this plan works.

Chapter Twenty Two

CONCLUSION

Incredible situations do happen even in times of when Gina and I had experienced great sorrow.

Out of nowhere my niece, Dr. Karen Heitzman (Dr. Jim's daughter) forwarded me a note in March 2008, from former patient, Joe Palmieri, whom I had removed a left ventricular aneurysm in 1969, and the rest is history. The response to the newspaper articles published in June 2008 has been amazing. Hence this book.

I have realized for some time no one living except myself is acquainted with the actual history and details of the beginning of open heart surgery in Syracuse, New York. It began at St. Joseph's Hospital to be exact and there are a number of important people who participated in this endeavor and they have never been credited or acknowledged.

Recording the incidents and people involved is very important. Without their efforts--my brother, patients, doctors, nurses, hospital workers, and in particular Sister Wilhelmina--this would never have materialized.

My brother had an endless number of friends, was extremely well liked and revered. He is sorely missed.

Brother Jim I hope you enjoyed it, I know where you are.

Although my open heart surgical career ended in 1972 I have been most fortunate in seeing the fulfillment of this dream. I have been truly blessed in spending the remaining years fulfilled in performing thoracic surgery and enjoying the unique and satisfying relationships with my patients.

There are still many unanswered questions as to the series of events during the birth of open heart surgery in Syracuse. I am at peace that I may never find the answers.

I hope you enjoyed my book; it has been a most painful process for me but healing and necessary to put closure. Thank you, Joe Palmieri!

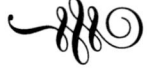

Chapter Twenty Three

ACKNOWLEDGEMENTS

Despite its divergent path, I had a wonderful medical career and am grateful to many individuals--unsung heroes and heroines--who were instrumental to either the establishment and development of the open heart program at St. Joseph's or to me personally in my private practice.

I'd like to acknowledge the following people:

In 1969, I was fortunate enough to hire a tremendous secretary, Rosemary Haller. She had worked in medical records at St. Joseph's. It was a privilege to employ her until my retirement in 1988. It would have been impossible to replace Rosemary as she was so talented. She was always fine appearing, bright, efficient, and punctual with the highest of principles. Patients loved her.

Dr. Jim's secretary, Mary DiMauro, worked for him more than 25 years, including the last phase of his career in industrial medicine. With his demise, Mary remained with this industrial group and held many responsible positions. She had many wonderful qualities and the ability to handle many situations and people simultaneously in a superb manner. She was always very supportive of my brother's widow.

Were it not for Dr. Paul Maglione, this book would never have been written. Paul is an excellent family physician in North Syracuse whom my brother and I have known and worked with for many years. He and Joe Palmieri are cousins and Joe consulted him in 1969 for a cardiac evaluation. This led to an immediate heart catheterization at St. Joseph's Hospital and subsequent open heart surgery. Paul was a strong supporter of the open heart program at St. Joseph's in its infancy and subsequently. He is an extremely caring and capable physician and one I have always enjoyed.

There was a recent write-up of him in our local newspaper highlighting his wonderful career.

A major early contributor to the heart surgery program and the cardiopulmonary laboratory was cardiologist Asher Black. He was a very colorful, animated fellow, well informed and a fine cardiologist. He supported Dr. Delmonico with closed heart surgery in the years before I arrived. His patients loved him.

Dr. Sam Schlamowitz was a board certified cardiologist and very academic. He, too, was a strong supporter of the new program. Several internists-cardiologists were great contributors from the onset. In addition to Dr. Jim, they included: Carl Austin, Ed Mullin, Jack O'Brien, Harry McKinnon, Bill Schiess, John Duggan, J.G. Fred Hiss, Charlie Hitchcock, John Dadey, and Murray Grossman. There were also out-of-town referring internists: R.J. Marilley and Fred Taylor of Watertown, and Bob Taylor and Joe Rowley of Auburn.

Without the following family physicians the program would never have succeeded: Ernie Carhart, Roger Daley, Tom Bishop, and Howard Platz from Minoa; Carl Marlow, John Merola, Paul Maglione, Howard Livingston, Armand Cincotta, Sam Paris from North Syracuse; Steve Cost, Jerry Stiner, Walter Sutherland, Joel Potash, Norman Lipton, Chuck Elliot, Marshall Fulmer, Tom Snyder, Norm Elitharp, Bill Fallon, Bob Walker, Joe Guerarra, Joe Birard from Syracuse; and pediatricians Chuck Needham, Ralph Prowda, Marty Ushkow, and Bob Shapiro.

My apologies for unintentionally excluding anyone.

Gene Morreale was a tremendous asset when he arrived at St. Joseph's Hospital. He was assigned to the record room, which was in shambles, and restored it to a top notch facility with dispatch and at the same time with a friendly, cheerful manner without irritation or confrontation at any time. This is indeed a most difficult task when dealing with physicians!

Gene was always very efficient, humble and task oriented. It was a pleasure to see him advance to assistant administrator and I was most disappointed when he was not appointed head administrator at St. Joseph's. We never socialized but I followed his career from a distance and was elated when he was appointed administrator of Oneida Hospital. It is gratifying to see someone of Gene's talents and capabilities to succeed to the top in an extremely competitive environment. He has the ingredients to advance even further.

George More was chief of operations at Syracuse Surgical. I first met him when he came to correct a problem with the Forrester heart-lung machine. I was so impressed that I recommended he become a full time hospital employee assigned to the open heart team.

Until that happened, Dr.Delmonico and I paid for his attendance at all open heart procedures because we felt his presence was instrumental to the smooth running of the machine, and thus, patient safety. Eventually the hospital paid for these services and he joined the staff. I encouraged George to become certified as an open heart perfusionist to operate the heart-lung. He recalls my bringing in a pile of books and articles on operating the machine along with two medical dictionaries to study for the exams. In 1974, George became a certified perfusionist, the only one at the time.

As previously mentioned, my brother knew the employees at St. Joseph's Hospital very well and almost daily had breakfast with the plumbers, painters, etc.--the pulse of the hospital. One of those regulars in a key position was the hospital's Director of Purchasing, Everett Price. He was a typical New Englander, accent and all, and loved spending time on the Cape in September when the summer visitors had gone. Everett was affable and very civic minded and had been the chief of the Dewitt Voluntary Fire Department for years. As a result, at the hospital he was usually affectionately called "Chief." I classify Everett as a true loyal hospital employee who could be completely trusted to support the hospital.

Dr. Richard Hehir has been our internist for many years and we consider him a very good friend and an excellent internist. His secretary, Sally, is pleasant, organized, and runs a tremendous office. It is amazing to see this solo practice care for such a large volume of patients and do it so personally.

The entire spectrum of medicine has changed so much but Dr. Hehir has maintained very high standards. Nowadays, it is unheard of for an internist to make house visits but Dick does this on occasion and recently visited my best friend, Bob Peet, who was ill at home. Both Bob and his wife, Joan, were impressed with Dick's worn out black leather bag, reminiscent of the "old country doc."

Only recently I learned that Dick volunteers at least once a week at the Poverello Health Center, part of the Franciscan Northside Ministries, which offers free health care for the indigent with no health insurance.

Dick is very proud of his two sons who are also doctors.

Dr. Harold Wanamaker another individual I greatly admired and respected. In the early 1970s, I underwent an ear operation for deafness from an inherited otosclerosis that previously afflicted my father. He and I are the only known family members with this. He was deaf ever since I can remember and this made it very difficult for my mother. Hearing aids were available but he would not use one. I discovered my hearing loss when making a trip west looking for possible relocation to do heart surgery in 1972. For the first time, I could not hear the ticking of my wrist watch in my right ear.

Soon after, I went to an ENT specialist whom I knew rather well. The diagnosis was made and surgery recommended. Otosclerosis involves a progressive fibrosis among the tiny three bones in the middle ear. In the procedure to correct it, a bone in the middle ear is removed and replaced with a tiny wire. This is fine, tedious surgery. I went through the procedure well and immediately could hear much better. I went home and vigorously worked out in the back yard when I experienced all kinds of noises and dizziness from the right ear. I consulted my surgeon, who responded, "Didn't I tell you to go home, rest and do nothing?" I did not hear him say that, if he did. Needless to say, I lost the entire hearing in the left ear and only a cochlear implant would help.

One of the previous interns at St. Joseph's Hospital, Dr. David Rodriguez, had started an ear, nose and throat residency at Upstate. I knew him very well and when he learned of my problem he advised me to consult Dr. Harold Wanamaker. Harold was a very busy and successful otolaryngologist in private practice and did his surgery at Crouse Memorial Hospital. I also learned that he was extremely busy, experienced, and successful with stapedectomy, the medical term for replacing this bone in the middle ear with a wire. He admitted me immediately and within two hours I was in the operating room. He explored the operative site, via the ear drum, hoping that the wire had displaced. Unfortunately it had not, and nothing more could be done. With my physical activity spinal fluid had leaked and the cranial nerve of the brain for hearing was permanently damaged.

I was so impressed with Harold Wanamaker. He cancelled everything and did an emergency exploration of my ear. Ever since, I have found him to be a most unusual giving person.

Not only was he an outstanding otolaryngologist, but he was truly a special human being. He has constantly been lauded, along with his wife, for community philanthropy and helping their fellow man. Much of this is in the newspapers; more is not. The moral of this story: go to the very best and never settle for less.

They have two sons, Hayes and John, both otolaryngologists who have worked with their father. Since Hal's retirement, I have been treated by both and found them to be very much like their dad.

I can't say enough about Jim Longo. When my internist, Dr. Dick Hehir advised me to see a cardiologist for further evaluation, unhesitatingly I requested Dr. Jim Longo. There are good reasons for this.

When active in thoracic surgery, I well recall a young LeMoyne College student working part time at St. Joseph's in the operating room as an operating room technician from between 1974 and 1977. His name was Jim Longo. Previously he had worked in the hospital kitchen for three years.

He frequently assisted me with minor procedures such as bronchoscopies and mediastinoscopies. He was always well-mannered, very interested, and efficient.

In the 1990s, while reviewing patient charts for the Peer Review Organization, I had occasion to review a number of Dr. Longo's charts from Crouse Irving Memorial Hospital. I never placed him as the Jim Longo from St. Joe's, but recognized that the quality of his charts, notes, etc., was outstanding. Shortly after, I learned of a Katie Longo in our son Jacob's kindergarten class but I did not put all the pieces together until a parent's meeting at school. There was Katie's dad, Dr. James Longo, my O.R. tech from the 1970s! We both enjoyed renewing acquaintances and recalled old times. He had graduated from LeMoyne in 1977 and Upstate Medical School in 1981. Needless to say, I complimented him on his meticulous charts. I also learned that he knew my brother from working as a medical student in the emergency room at St. Joe's where EJ was chief. He related that once while he was working in the emergency room and my brother learned it was his wedding anniversary he gave him a gift certificate to Julie's restaurant, a favorite on James Street.

When my brother was seriously ill in 1996 and hospitalized at Crouse Memorial, Jim Longo learned of this and, although not his physician, quietly arranged for my brother to be transferred immediately into a private room for his remaining few days of life. Shortly after E.J.'s death he wrote me a most caring letter expressing his and his wife's heartfelt feelings about my brother and their enrollment of him into the perpetual membership of The Marianist Spiritual Alliance. I have cherished this from him.

Needless to say when I personally needed a cardiologist I sought out Jim, who has cared for me in a superior manner. Our children continued to be in the same class through high school and graduated together.

I would remiss to exclude Dr. Longo's associates and office staff. This office is outstanding in all respects including medical expertise, friendliness and concern. I have known Dr. Bill Berkery for at least 10 years socially and later professionally. He epitomizes the ideal physician.

I consider Dr. Jack Nicholson, a colon surgeon, as a friend and one of the most capable physicians I have met. He has cared for my family and close friends in very fine fashion.

Urologist Dr. Buz Roberts is very highly rated in all respects as a physician and person and I have appreciated his care and concern over the years. He was early in the use of robotic surgery.

My wife and I have used Wegman's pharmacy in Dewitt for many years and have been extremely pleased. However the entity is comprised of specific humans and this is where the personal touch is so important. We have recently enjoyed a relationship with a young pharmacist, Vicki Stenuf. She has the necessary ingredients for success anywhere with her appearance, knowledge and warm concerned manner. Such care leaves one with much satisfaction and confidence.

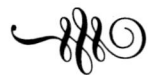

ADDENDUM

In June, 2008, the Syracuse *Post-Standard* published a beautiful front-page article, "To Touch Hearts," that chronicled the story of former Joe Palmieri, our recent reunion in Ithaca, and touched on some of the history of my early open heart cases in Syracuse.

The response to the article was overwhelming; I received letters, emails, and telephone calls from patients I hadn't heard from in many years. Their outpouring was truly what motivated this memoir.

The following is a sample of those remarks:

Dear: Dr. Heitzman:

We first met in your office at the State Tower Building on April 11th, 1966 for consultation regarding mitral valve surgery at the request of Dr. R.J. Marilley Jr. of Watertown, New York. You were in complete agreement with Dr. Marilley that I had significant mitral valvicular stenosis. Surgery was scheduled at St Joseph's hospital on Wednesday May 18th, 1966 and Dr. Goffredo Gensini did a Cardiac catheterization that revealed a tight (85% closed) mitral stenosis. Surgery was performed on May 18th when I underwent mitral valve commissurotomy. This surgery was performed by you, Dr. Ernrst Delmonico and staff while Sister Laurine operated the Mayo-Gibbons pumps. Your brother, Dr. Ed Heitzman, was the cardiologist that administered my daily medical course. I was discharged on June 1st, 1966 on a low sodium diet with no heart medication

Heart fibrillation was a complication for five months but return to near normal. The valve was free of calcium and my rheumatic heart disease inactive. I did return to work seven months later on the same position I had left for surgery. At that time I was 28 years old, married and the father of three young boys: two preteens and the youngest one was five. My youngest son celebrated the successful surgery by telling his friends that he would not have to get a new daddy, because his daddy did not die.

My health continued to improve and life returned to near normal for 10 years. I had been promoted to a salaried management position, completed several course of higher education and was well on my way to a good career when restenosis occurred after a very successful mitral commissurotomy. On December 30th, 1975 I was admitted to The Carthage Area Hospital for congestive heart failure. On January, 19th, 1976 I was again admitted to St. Joseph's Hospital, Syracuse for cardiac catheterization by Dr. Goffredo Gensini, by then Director of Cardiovascular Laboratory and Research Department, which revealed severe restenosis.

I did after consultations with several doctors delay this on the advice of Dr. Sunder Iqbal, until October 17th, 1978 in hopes that replacement valve would be improved. On October 17th, 1978 mitral valve replacement was implanted in my heart at St. Joseph's Hospital by Dr. Donald B. Effler and Dr. Biosia (not sure of the spelling). This valve lasted over 20 years when scar tissue grew over barrel and again closed the valve. This was another 20 year period of success, career advancement, goal of seeing my children reach adulthood and retirement at the age of 55.

On November 4th, 1998 Mitral valve replacement (St. Jude Medical) was implanted in my heart at St. Joseph's Hospital by Dr. Ahmad Nazem.

On September 17th, 1996 I had cardiac pacemaker implanted and on September 15, 2003 it was replaced. Both at St. Jude by Dr. Ashraf and Dr. Khan at Carthage Area Hospital.

I was also admitted to St. Joseph's Hospital for acute endocarditis from October 25th. 1983 to November 9th, 1983 by Dr. Sunder Iqbal.

Life has always been good, but never easy, challenge is a great motivator and I believe I was determined to accept greater challenges after my health was restored by your dedicated services to me and my family I think that as a great-grandfather at 71 years of age that I can say with great sincerity, THANK YOU Dr. Heitzman for a good job well done, with more understanding of the value of life and life's values. Some of the events that have occurred in the last 42 years since 1966, that would not have been possible for me without successful surgery when open heart surgery was first advancing through the pioneer stage are celebrating my 53rd wedding anniversary with my wife Carol, seeing our children reach adulthood, seeing our 9 grandchildren reach adulthood, complete further education, enjoying our four great grandchildren with two more on the way this spring, traveling to 48 of the 50 states, traveling to six European countries, vacationing in Hawaii, enjoying hunting and fishing trips to Montana, Texas, Georgia, Michigan, Hudson bay and other destinations with my sons, excellent career and retirement at the age of 55. We reside in upstate New York for 6 months and Southern Florida for six months for the past 16 years. Thank you for the opportunity to enjoy these events and thousands of other events and occasions.

I encourage you to write a book and pledge to purchase the first autographed copy you have for sale. I would travel to Syracuse to meet with you for lunch, dinner, or just for a conversation about the last 42 years in both of our lives at your convenience and a place of your choice.

Thank you,

Robert F.

Dear Dr. Heitzman,

After seeing the article in the newspaper about your career, it took me back to the spring of 1962. That was the year that you and Dr. Ernest Delmonico, Jr. performed open heart surgery on me and changed my life forever.

I had been born a blue baby (that is what they called it in 1938). My mother was told by the doctors that I would not survive to adulthood. I visited many clinics throughout my childhood and was told the same thing. When I became pregnant with my first child, I was informed that I would not make it through the delivery. I had a very good Primary Care Physician that helped me through the delivery of my daughter and then referred me to Dr. Asher Black.

Dr Black sent me to St. Joseph's hospital for a Heart Catheter (Anagram) and then set up a meeting with two surgeons, you and Dr. Delmonico, Jr.

It was a very frightening time, knowing that the procedure was so new. Frightening as it was, I realized that I was becoming weaker, and that my only hope of seeing my daughter grow up was to go forward with the surgery.

At that time an ice blanket was used to bring down my temperature for the procedure. After the surgery, I awoke in severe pain, but with each day it became more bearable.

After being home a few weeks, I experienced severe chest pain. My husband rushed me to the hospital. I still remember seeing you all dressed up, probably leaving a party, to check on me. It turned out to be inflamed scar tissue. I was so grateful that you took the time to see me at the hospital and put my anxieties to rest.

The weeks and months that followed brought a healthy vibrance that I had never experienced in all my life. I had energy, an appetite, and hope for a future.

I went on to have two more children, eight grandchildren and two great grandchildren. It has been a little over forty six years and still no problems with the surgery.

I want you to know how much I appreciate your dedication. Your skilled hands have given me a full life.

Thank You
Sincerely,
Joyce BC

My name is MJ K. and I want to share with you two very significant stories of people Dr. Heitzman has helped so that they could bless my life with love and happiness.

I first would like to tell you the story of my father, AK. He smoked an average of two packs of cigarettes a day and acquired cancer in his left lung. I was 7 years old and don't remember too much of what led up to the surgery, but I certainly can relive for you what happened after. My father's lung was removed on Friday. I made my First Communion on Sunday and the hospital allowed me to go to the hospital in my dress and veil to see my Dad. At the time they did not allow children that age to visit, but made an exception because his prognosis was extremely grim. Whoever began the examination decided that because of the seriousness of it and the amount of cancer, my Father would not live more than a few days after surgery (if he survived it at all).

Dr. Heitzman had other plans, Thank God!! He said that would not be the case if he had anything to do with it. He said there was a new procedure that could be used, so he partnered with a doctor named DeMong. My Mother told me later that my father stopped breathing while on the operating table for about five minutes.
Dr. Heitzman told me it was a very special day because I had received Jesus for the first time and it was special also because it was the first day of my father's recovery. He said God gave him back to us and he was sure God would heal him totally.

Dr. Heitzman visited every single day, sometimes twice a day and oversaw his recovery. I thank God for his determination to save my Dad. That man that was supposed to live just a few days, lived 15 years after that lung was removed. I had my Dad in my life to see me grow and have a child of my own. He never did stop smoking entirely (only every 40 days of lent) but would begin after Easter Sunday. So the inevitable happened and he got cancer in the only lung he had left when I was 22 years old. I lost him in the eighth month of my pregnancy.

If it weren't for the knowledge, extreme dedication and compassion of Dr. Heitzman, I would have been a 7-year old girl going to her father's funeral. Words cannot express my appreciation and gratitude to the man who has exemplified what the medical profession should be. It's wonderful to have gotten good grades in medical school, and it's wonderful to have had a successful residency, it is even wonderful to begin practice and please patients-----but it is so much more.

Dr. Heitzman truly appreciated the gift God gave him, to be a talented surgeon, but he gave so much more to every one of his patients. He gave his love and his caring and heartfelt compassion. He made my family feel like he believed my Dad was as important as we thought he was and offered inexhaustible energy to insure his quality of life would be restored to him and all of us as well.

I remember my Dad and Mom discussing him from time to time and saying "there will never be another doctor to measure up to Dr. George Heitzman". My Mother was a very religious woman and remembered him in her novenas and rosaries right up until the time she died (21 years later).

As if this story isn't poignant enough and wasn't enough for me to cherish knowing this remarkable man, he gave me another gift of a precious individual in my life. My best friend, J.

In 1960 a young eighteen year old girl name JB was in a horrible car accident and was extremely injured. She was taken to St. Joe's and as she puts it, "was tortured with every test known to man", her stomach in her chest, in excruciating pain and thinking she was going to die any minute.

She said a couple of days after she was admitted, a man walked into her room. She tells me all she could think was how beautiful his eyes were, how they almost spoke to her. This man, Dr. Heitzman said she was the talk of the hospital. He said he thought he could help her, would she let him. She said yes, and from that moment on, she had hope for the first time since she was in the hospital. He said he needed time to check all the tests that had been done and then decide where to go from there.

J. told me there was a horrible snowstorm and cars couldn't get up the hill to St. Joe's. Did that stop Dr. Heitzman? Absolutely not, she told me he parked his car and walked the rest of the way so he could check on her. He promised and didn't want to disappoint her.

As you may have guessed, he operated, took her lung and got her well. She married, had four children, went through a number of very serious female operations and is still going strong at 68 years old. She lives in Florida now, so it is difficult for us to see each other, but we speak regularly and still to this day mention her love, Dr. George Heitzman, the man who saved her life.

I am 65 years old now, quite a few years past 7. I see him in church at Sunday Mass and still thank God for the talent this man gave to so many people for so many years. When our pastor, Father Kevin says "Reflect on how you have seen Jesus" I look at Dr. Heitzman and think,

"This wonderful man has brought Jesus to me each time I looked at my Dad and saw him hold my baby daughter and each time I talk to my best friend Joyce".

One of the many gifts I have received from God is this man, and I pray that our Father bestows a wonderful crown to shine brightly in Heaven on the head of a man who loved his God, his patients, and was a shining example of what all Christians should be.

Dr. Heitzman, what a humble man you are. Thank you for all you've done. I'm sure all the patients that you have given a second chance at life would say the same. There are many compliments on this page for the person you are and what you have accomplished. It sounds like well-deserved praise.

~ L.

Very nice article. And Dr. Heitzman, if you are reading this, write that book!! At least you know you will sell one copy (to me).

~ A.E.

What a heart warming story.
I'll buy one too.

~ L.

Hi Maureen-

Congratulations to you on such a great article in regard to Dr. George Heitzman. Just like so many others, Dr. Heitzman touched our family's heart too. It was 21 years ago that my mother-in-law had lung cancer. It all happened so fast. I don't know, other than by the Grace of God, that we were fortunate enough to have Dr. Heitzman as my mother-in-law's surgeon. He sucessfully removed a portion of her lung and she has been cancer free since. Dr. Heitzman answered so many questions for our family, and I'm sure we asked him the same ones over and over again. Our family was blessed to have a surgeon who is not only the best in his field, but has some wonderful "bedside" manners. We will never forget the times he sat on the edge of her bed and took her hand to reassure her (and us) that she was going to be alright. The best thing about it was, he knew she would be alright, he was not "just saying" it. He always knew what was going on, good or bad, and always knew just how to explain it. In the years to come after my mother-in-law's recovery, we kept in touch with Dr. Heitzman and his wife Gina.

Dr. Heitzman gave us a gift that day we met him, the gift of himself. He helped us through another family member's passing, and so many other medical "emergencies" throughout the years. He has given us his family's friendship. He is someone special that our impressionable teenage son looks up to, respects and admires. How fortunate we are to have had the Heitzmans in our lives. We have learned so much from Dr. Heitzman and his wife. They are both amazingly beautiful people and I hope they know just how much they mean to us.

Thank you for your time Maureen.

The B. Family

Dear Maureen,

I just wanted to write and let you know what a fabulous job you did on the article on Dr. George Heitzman. I met George in 1983 socially but then in 1985 chose to have him operate on me for a collapsed lung. Since then my husband and I have consulted with George for every medical problem we have had over the years and we have had a few more than we would have liked. We have become very good friends with both Gina and George and think the world of both of them. It was heartwarming to see a tribute to a man who is so deserving of it. Thank you again for printing this so others could see what a wonderful man he is.

Linda E.

Doctor George Heitzman,

It was so heart warming to read that lovely article about you and now to hear from you via this email after so many years, it is great to know you too are well.

There was an ESM Student that I know that had the same punma thorax (obviously I am not a doctor nor can I spell what I had...) but in talking about the procedure I went through with him, it was completely different that what little he had to go through in this day and age. I actually took my 14-year old son to our family doctors last week as he was complaining of pains in a region similar to what

I seem to remember; and he has shot up about 4-6" in the last couple of months.....x-rays did not show anything though.

Small world, I reside in East Syracuse-Minoa School district with wife and two boys, and am proud to be serving on their School Board of Education.

If there are any passages or names you want to use in your book referencing me, please feel free. As well as to contact me for anything.....

All the best in your retirement,

Kevin C. B.

Dear Maureen:

I read your article in yesterday's paper about the great surgeon Dr. George Heitzman. I was so pleased to see he was so well at his age and still so good looking.

The reason it brought tears to my eyes was that it brought back memories for me when I was 18-19 years old. That was the first time I met Dr. Heitzman at St. Joe's and his partner Dr. Delmonico because I worked under Sister Mary Letitia in the medical records department which used to be on the side of the emergency room at that time. I worked for her off and on for several summers while I attended Maria Regina and Lemoyne College well in the early 70's.

During that time I was a medical transcriptionist and transcribed all the surgeries done at St. Joe's. Among those were the famous heart surgeries done by that heart team. I was very proud to have transcribed the ones done during the summers I worked there. Some of the operations were 12 hours long and I still remember the pride I felt when I was asked to be exclusively the one who did the transcriptions for that team, requested by Dr. Heitzman. I was told that the reason was that they liked my work and my spelling. I had my training at Maria Regina and was pursuing a degree as a medical assistant. I went on to pursue a different occupation and am now a insurance agent but my hobby is still medicine. If he ever needs any help (proofreading, typing) as I am an old, old secretary when he starts his book have him contact me.

When I read that he had some of the actual operations I wondered if he was looking at the ones I typed under the name of (MAP).

It was amazing the lives he was able to save and the history he made for St. Joe's in those early years. It was very suspenseful working there as we all monitored the surgeries he performed and the outcome; in those days we would enter the cafeteria on the 2nd floor, going by the specimen room which I never failed to stop and look at the jars, and eat lunch with the surgeons who came down with the same clothes they operated on that day.

Dr. Heitzman was a very humble and religious man that simply walked the halls making history as a miracle worker, very oblivious to his skill calling it "luck."

Please give him my sincere regards.

Marie V.

Approximately 21 years ago, Dr. Heitzman saved the life of a family member. It was lung cancer. This doctor is not only brilliant, but a caring, warm and an exceptionally beautiful individual. Over the years he has kept in touch with our family. He also helped us through some very difficult times with another family member in which he was not the provider of care. However, he always took time for that frantic phone call at any time, day or night. Let the works of Dr. Heitzman be an example and inspiration to all. Thank you Dr. Heitzman for the skill in your hands, the warmth of your heart, and for giving our family the opportunity to love our mom a while longer. God Bless you and Gina.

~ A.

Dr. Heitzman,
As an RN at St. Joe's, I remember you well, and you too, Gina. What a great story. I can still recall your soft spoken way as well as your expertise. I'm sure a lot of people from St. Joseph's will be buying that book when you get it written.

~ S.

This is the most beautiful and uplifting article I have ever read, thank you for publishing it. Dr. Heitzman, you look the same as I remember you from 30 years ago when I worked with you at the hospital. You were always very nice and cheerful and always had extra time to spend with your sick patients (wish we had more like you), always lifting spirits and reassuring. Yes please write your book, I'd love to purchase it.
May God reward you and your family with the best of health. God Bless.

~ H.

Maureen - I have just read your article about Dr. George Heitzman, a man I will never forget as well. It was Dr. Heitzman back in 1982 who performed surgery on me as a 25 year old. My lungs collapsed several times and he recommended surgery to repair this. Knock on wood, but I have been fine now for almost 26 years now.

Is there an email address for Dr. Heitzman that you could share with me; as I too would like to reach out and thank him as well? His picture looks so much like the Doc who took great care of me years ago.

Thanks, and again....great article Maureen

Kevin B.

Maureen:

I would imagine you are getting a number of responses to your article on Doctor Heitzman. I too have a Very full and happy life due in a large part to St. Joes. Surely I'm living a lot longer and healthier because of Doctors Heitzman, Delmonico and Gensiene and their team back in 1959. Pretty wild to think back, at 9 I was told I was sick, (did not feel sick) would be in the hospital for 2-3 weeks, miss a month and a half of school (cool)etc. and now I'm 58, have 2 grown kids, very grateful to my parents and that team of very competent folks. I would like to send my thanks on to Doctor Heitzman and ask a question or two.

If there is a way you could send this on or recommend a way to communicate with Dr. Heitzman I would greatly appreciate it.

Thanks again,

Mike M.

Note: See enclosed photo of him walking into St. Joe's Hospital with his mother for the heart surgery in 1960.

I have had the privilege to observe my husband in the operating room, in the office and at home. The adjectives that I can use to best describe him are respect and love by both his patients and the nurses and health care providers that he has worked with.

My husband is very humble and shy. His enormous contributions to humanity are private. He will minimize his impact.

He performed the first open heart surgery case at St. Joseph's Hospital and surely in Syracuse. He performed the first pacemaker implant and mediastinoscopy procedure.

What separates him from other fine physicians is his continued interest in helping people whether it is family, friends, or past patients and even their families well into his retirement of almost 20 years. He will never turn anyone away to make a recommendation, a referral or call a colleague on behalf of a person in need.

He is not a politician and has always avoided the limelight. I remember when he operated on Bishop Harrison on Good Friday at St. Joseph's there were reporters and camera crews waiting for him outside the hospital. He exited through the back door of the hospital to avoid publicity.

It would be impossible for me to note all of the responses, gifts etc. that he has received through the years from grateful people. Everyone was taken care of irrespective of health insurance or not.

We met a police officer who worked with my husband at St. Joe's as an EMT and said to me "I watched your husband save lives with his bare hands, I have the utmost respect for him."

I have observed his relationships with interns and residents through the years. He takes them under his wing and becomes a father figure to them. Two especially that come to mind are Dr. Amilcar Barreto presently living in San Antonio, Texas and Dr. Roberto Canto, a successful physician in San Juan, Puerto Rico. Dr. Canto stated to my husband "you were kind to me when no one else was." I have been most fortunate to be married to this man.

Joe Palmieri kindled something in him and hence this book. I think for him its been an incredible life review and it's a validation.

Sincerely,
Gina H.